Ad

& *5 St*

*"**5 Steps to a Hollywood A-List Smile** will encourage anyone to take care of their dental health and to feel better about themselves for doing it. It's a great inspiration towards self-love and creating a confidence within yourself."*

~ Common, Grammy award-winning rapper and actor

"Thank you for aiding in my smile. I love and appreciate your work and dedication!"

~ Paula Abdul, American Idol host and Grammy award-winning singer

"Dr. Austin is just what dentistry needed! She is warm, friendly and knows what is best for her patients. There are no worries when sitting in her chair! I am happy that she is responsible for my platinum smile!"

~ Legendary Rapper Slick Rick

*"You don't have to be a celebrity to get a red carpet smile. **5 Steps to a Hollywood A-List Smile** reveals the celebrity dental secrets and procedures that EVERYONE can use to smile like the stars and feel more confident from the very first page!"*

~ Mickey Burns, NYC TV Host

*"As my personal dentist for many years now, Dr. Austin has shared many helpful tips on how to keep my smile camera ready. From beginning to end, **5 Steps to a Hollywood A-List Smile** brings home the message of how important it is to have a healthy smile and how it can not only make you look better, but also give you the confidence to make power moves in life, to attract the opposite sex and, more importantly, keep you in good health overall."*

~ Malik Yoba, Actor

"This book is a must-read for anyone who has always wanted a Hollywood smile but didn't know how to begin the process and their options. ***5 Steps to a Hollywood A-List Smile*** *tells you everything you need to know to get the smile of your dreams!"*

~ Natalie Vavricka, Associate Editor QualityHealth.com

*"**5 Steps to a Hollywood A-List Smile** is a priceless resource guide from award-winning cosmetic dentists to the stars, Dr. Catrise Austin."*

~ Laurie N. Robinson, CEO and Founder of Corporate Counsel Women of Color

*"**5 Steps to a Hollywood A-List Smile** is definitely not just your typical self-help book. Dr. Catrise Austin is a skilled professional who is very pleasant and down-to-earth and her '5 Steps' will provide you with the information you need regardless of your profession."*

~ Cheryl Smith, Executive Editor for *Dallas Weekly*

"To sum up VIP Smiles, it's 'Dentistry Done with Love!' I'm proud to be her client for the past 10 years and also her friend. Keep us smiling!"

~ Godfrey, Actor/Comedian

"As a celebrity photographer, I have the pleasure of working with and showcasing the images of today's biggest stars. A beautiful smile is one of the first things that I notice in my photographs. It doesn't matter if you're wearing designer clothes, the finest jewels, or how trendy your hairstyle is, if your smile is not presentable it can really make or break your image! Dr. Austin's ***5 Steps to a Hollywood A-list Smile*** *is a consumer guide that will definitely help you get a picture-perfect smile."*

~ Johnny Nunez, Photography By Johnny Nunez

As Seen On *Good Morning America, Discovery Health, & BET*

5 Steps to a Hollywood A-List Smile:

How the Stars Get That Perfect Smile – And How You Can, Too!

By Dr. Catrise Austin

www.vipsmiles.com

with Rusty Fischer

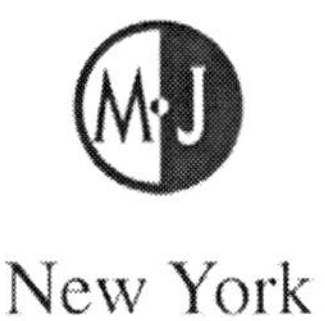

New York

5 Steps to the Hollywood A-List Smile

How the Stars Get That Perfect Smile and How You Can Too!

ISBN 978-1-60037-644-3

Library of Congress Control Number:

MORGAN · JAMES
THE ENTREPRENEURIAL PUBLISHER

Morgan James Publishing, LLC
1225 Franklin Ave., STE 325
Garden City, NY 11530-1693
Toll Free 800-485-4943
www.MorganJamesPublishing.com

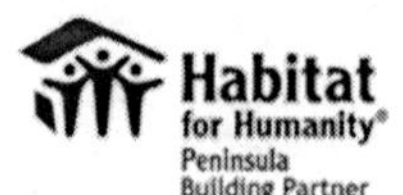

Acknowledgments

So many people go into the creation of a published book; I hardly know where to start. But this list of A-list friends, family, colleagues and mentors has truly inspired me throughout the years and made this book possible. To them all, my undying love and appreciation:

First to Michele Austin, my mother; my rock. We've grown together in many ways and I thank God constantly for providing me with the most supportive mother in the world; the type of mother that people *dream* of having! Thank you for always being there for me and believing in me, especially in those times that I didn't believe in myself.

To the rest of the Austins (Alicia & Elijiah, Uncle Willie, Aunt Angie) and extended family, thank you for your support and encouragement to live my dream. Special thanks to Grandma Carlean and my late Grandpa Whilmon Austin for encouraging my education and helping me get through college. (Oh, and for the banana pudding and collard greens, too!)

Dr. Oscar Wright, you changed my life right when I needed it by encouraging me to improve my smile. You inspired me to become a dentist and for that I am forever thankful. I now help others the way you helped me!

Mr. Mike Larson, thank you for giving me a chance and trusting me with your patients in high school. You were my first example of an entrepreneur. I learned the art of customer service, empathy and compassion from YOU.

To my closest friend since high school, Darlene; we made it! It has been a pleasure growing up with you. You've been by my side since we both got teased in high school about our teeth and for studying too much. I couldn't ask for a better friend. You are the smartest person I know and you truly inspire me to keep rising to the top.

Thanks to the staff, my fellow classmates, and alumni at The University of Maryland Dental School for your support over the years. Special thanks to Billie Brown Gardner for the countless boxes of tissues that I used in your office and, most importantly, for encouraging me to press on in dental school.

Special thanks to Dr. Albert Thompson and Dr. Karen Gear for being my mentors over the years and helping me start my dental practice, VIP Smiles, in New York City. There is no way that this dream would've come true without your guidance.

Special thanks to Renee Foster; thank you for igniting my career!

To Charles Williams of WEG Media, thank you for managing all of my technical needs and keeping me current with the times.

To the late Isaac Hayes; I miss you. You took me under your wing and supported me from the start of my career. You opened up my world and exposed me to people, places and things that have truly enriched my life.

Common, thank you for many years of support and friendship.

Mona Scott Young of Monami Entertainment, thanks for always having my back!

Janice "Mama" Combs, you mean the world to me.

The biggest thanks to all that helped give birth to my "baby" – *5 Steps to a Hollywood A-List Smile.* Raoul Davis, thank you for dedicating your time, knowledge and years of experience. My writing partner, Rusty Fischer, you are amazing and made this project seem like a breeze. My editor, Hanna Rubin, you're the best! Jimique aka JP Justice, you were such a tremendous help in helping me finish this project. Your innovative ideas and spirit inspires me to keep pressing on.

Last but never least, to all of my patients at VIP Smiles who travel from near and far, thanks for allowing me to serve you for over 10 years. There would be no me without you.

Contents

Author's Note

Dentistry changed my life as a teenager and I am forever grateful. Has dentistry changed your life? Has a smile enhancement helped you feel more confident? Helped you land a dream job? Helped you attract your mate? Share your story or thoughts on www.hollywoodalistsmiles.com.

Not only is it important in my daily practice to give the gift of a smile, but also to give back to the community and our world. There are so many organizations and people that helped me climb the ladder of success from high school to the present that I feel it is my duty to give as others have given to me.

I've listed my favorite non-profits below; each are truly changing the lives of many people and making a difference in our world by serving and training women and youth. A portion of the proceeds from the sale of this book will be donated to these organizations. You can learn more about these organizations on www.hollywoodalistsmiles.com or their respective websites.

Dress for Success

The mission of Dress for Success is to promote the economic independence of disadvantaged women by providing professional attire, a network of support and the career development tools to help women thrive in work and in life. Founded in New York City in 1997, Dress for

Success is an international not-for-profit organization offering services designed to help our clients find jobs and remain employed. Each Dress for Success client receives one suit when she has a job interview and can return for a second suit or separates when she finds work.

While we may be best known for providing suits to women, it is our employment retention programs that are the cornerstone of the organization. To meet the need for services that would help women both find and keep jobs, we established the Professional Women's Group (PWG) program, which offers women ongoing support as they successfully transition into the workforce, build thriving careers and prosper in the mainstream workplace. Dress for Success relies on the financial contributions, in-kind donations and volunteer efforts of individuals and companies around the world who are committed to helping women take charge of their lives. For more information, visit www.dressforsuccess.org.

Smiles for Success

The mission of Smiles for Success is to offer cost-free dental care to women graduates of accredited job readiness and placement programs or other community-based agencies thus helping those who are helping themselves. Smiles for Success is affiliated with numerous job readiness programs in over 30 states. The dental care offered is meant to be a short-term solution to those who need treatment unavailable to them through government programs or traditional insurance as they move from welfare to the working world. Smiles for Success, however, does not provide complete cosmetic smile makeovers. Smiles For Success programs also work in partnership with the aforementioned training programs, which have accredited and successful records in training and placing women in jobs. In addition, each Smiles For Success local area program works in conjunction with a clothing agency to outfit the potential candidate with suitable clothing for their interviews. For more information, visit www.smilesforsuccess.org.

Hope's Voice International

Hope's Voice International is an HIV and AIDS organization committed to promoting the education, prevention and the end of stigma of HIV and AIDS to young adults. Hope's Voice International aims to empower ambassadors and speakers--young adults living with HIV or AIDS--to be leaders in educating their communities and being catalysts for change. Hope's Voice International uses open dialogue and peer-to-peer education through the *Does HIV Look Like Me?* program presented by speakers at educational institutions and producing the *Does HIV Look Like Me?* international campaign with ambassadors in communities and countries around the globe. They send the crucial message: HIV and AIDS do not discriminate. At Hope's Voice International we aim to raise awareness and help young adults create the social change that is needed to end this epidemic and the stigma associated with it. For more information, visit www.hopesvoice.org and www.doeshivlooklikeme.org.

About This Book

"You're never fully dressed without a smile."

~ Martin Charnin

One of the earliest things my patients ask me when they sit in my chair for the very first time is, "What, exactly, is an A-List Smile?"

I always answer the same way, "You'll know it when you see one."

I'm not trying to be funny or flip; having an A-List Smile is kind of like being cool – hard to define but instantly recognizable the minute you see it. That's because having an A-List Smile is more than just whitening your teeth, having them shaped better or even straightening your teeth; with enough time and money just about anyone can do that.

An A-List Smile is as much a feeling as it is a filling; it is equal parts dentistry and psychology. That's because the mouth and the mind often go hand in hand. Better yet, smiling seems to be one of the cheapest, quickest and most efficient ways of having more confidence.

Actor, comedian and good friend Godfrey put it bluntly when he told me recently, "It's very important to have a nice smile in entertainment because your smile is one of the most important features. When you talk, people are always looking at your mouth. If your teeth are all jacked up, it's not a good look. So it's important to represent yourself with a good smile. Even if you ain't gotta dime, you at least, with nice teeth, look like you do!"

According to David Rogers, author of *How to Have Great Self*

Confidence, "Positive thinking is central to developing self confidence… smiling is simple, free, and something we all can do. Is your natural expression a smile or a frown? Observe other people – which ones look confident and at ease with the world? If you go around with a frown you may find you're too serious to let others near you! So smile – even if there is no reason to smile."

Your smile doesn't just boost your confidence; it can even boost your sex appeal! Just ask Karina Smirnoff from the hit show *Dancing with the Stars*, who recently said, "A smile speaks a thousand words. Having clean, white teeth can make your smile absolutely beautiful. As a professional dancer, confidence is very important and my smile helps me feel not only more confident, but sexy, too."

We all know this one basic fact to be true: when you look better, you feel better.

The beautiful part of that truism is that "better" is in the eye of the beholder. You don't have to look like someone else, be famous or hold yourself up to someone else's standards of beauty to feel good about yourself. I've worked on famous mouths like those of Paula Abdul, actor Kevin Sorbo, model/actress Eva Pigford, New York Jet's running back Leon Washington, rapper/actor Common, playwright Sarah Jones, and singers Isaac Hayes and Toni Braxton, but you don't have to be famous to want an A-List Smile. Looking better can be about you from the start; it doesn't have to be about looking like someone else.

That's why it's so hard to define an A-List Smile; it's different for everybody. But I know it when I see it. Some people think having a whiter smile makes it A-List; others want their teeth straightened; some think that having a metal-free mouth makes it A-List. That's why I take each patient on a mouth-by-mouth basis. It's also why I wrote ***5 Steps to a Hollywood A-List Smile**: How the Stars Get That Perfect Smile – and How You Can, Too!*

We may never meet in person, but I still want to help you achieve an A-List Smile no matter where you live. So by writing the first-ever self-help guidebook to getting an A-List Smile, I can walk you through the process step-by-step.

5 steps, to be exact…

Rating Your Smile: *A-List or D-List?*

Let's face it; in our beauty-conscious society, one of the first things people notice about you is your smile. It's your greeting card, your business card, your resume and your facial "mood ring" all in one. Over the course of my career I've discovered that helping people rate their smiles has helped them come to smart decisions about what they need to succeed.

So one of my first steps in this book is to help you gauge your A-List Smile using the age-old Hollywood ratings system to assess it. This includes:

1. **The "A-List" Smile (4 Stars – ****):** This is the Hollywood, red carpet ready smile that, just like the stars, you're proud to leave home with. It's the type of smile that makes people stop you on the street to compliment you on your smile and even ask you about your dentist. People with A-List smiles know it – and are not afraid to share with the world how confident and beautiful they feel.
2. **The "B-List" Smile (3 Stars – ***):** Although the B-List smile may have a *few* minor flaws, it is a smile that still manages to be presentable. It may not be a smile that is red-carpet ready, but with a little bit of tweaking using the latest cosmetic dentistry and general maintenance, this smile has the potential to become A-List!
3. **The "C-List" Smile (2 Stars – **):** If it's been awhile since someone complimented you on your smile, chances are you've fallen straight off the A-List, sailed past the "B-List" category and are stuck somewhere on the C-List; not quite the best but not quite the worst, either.
4. **The "D-List" Smile (1 Star – *):** This is a smile you'd rather wear at home; a mouth you feel insecure about anywhere but inside your own living room or home theater. Not to worry; *5 Steps to a Hollywood A-List Smile* can help.

The beauty of my 4-star rating system is that, just like an A-List Smile, it depends on who's doing the rating. In other words, it's not up to ME to tell YOU what your smile looks like; that's why it's called a "self" assessment. But it IS my job to help you understand the pros and cons of each type of smile – and what can be done to rectify your current smile **if you so desire**.

In fact, that's where *5 Steps to a Hollywood A-List Smile* was born...

5 Steps to a Hollywood A-List Smile

My name is Dr. Catrise Austin and I am a busy Manhattan dentist with a thriving private practice catering to some of New York City's most elite clientele. In a field traditionally dominated by men, I had to break many gender as well as racial boundaries by establishing my own ground with innovative operations and a unique business strategy that caters to Manhattan's entertainment leaders. In 1998, I opened an office under the banner "VIP Smiles," a modern dental practice that boasts an impressive loyal following, including some of the warmest smiles in the entertainment industry.

In March of 2007 I was asked by Aquafresh to be their traveling spokesperson for the newly launched Aquafresh White Trays over the counter teeth whitening system. In that capacity I have appeared at a variety of venues in Miami, Chicago, New York and Los Angeles on behalf of Aquafresh and the White Trays product line.

In addition, *The Discovery Health Channel*, *The Queen Latifah Show* and *The Ricki Lake Show* have all called on my services over the years. When *Essence*, *Glamour* or *Self* magazine needs a go-to dental expert with her fingers on the pulse of the entertainment industry, they call on me – as they have numerous times in the past.

I've been a guest expert on radio programs across the nation speaking about the importance of dental health, and I frequently make public speaking appearances to spread the message that "anyone can have an A-List Smile." Throughout the entertainment industry as well as communities across the nation, I am cultivating a reputation as a designer of great smiles.

But you don't have to live in Manhattan or be a movie star to utilize my services. With *5 Steps to a Hollywood A-List Smile* I share for the first time a wealth of advice on not just what dental products and services are available on the market today but just how much they can help create a brand new you.

People often think of the cosmetic changes that come from a brand new smile, but they rarely stop to appreciate the personal changes that come as well. I have helped many, many patients over the years become more confident, capable and happy people by letting them "grow into their smiles" and truly understand what it means to be satisfied with your appearance.

How we look has so much to do with how we feel these days. Right or wrong, looking good really does make us feel good – and what's wrong with that? If I can do one thing with this book it will be to help you be happier with how you look, whether that means a little work or a lot. When it comes to how you feel about your smile, you have choices, but you need to be honest with yourself. No one else can make those decisions – or those changes – for you. This book will help you come to the right choice for YOU.

My goal is to guide you on how you can make your mouth as special and pleasing as it can be. This way you can quit worrying about your teeth and start living your life. And trust me, if there's anyone who knows about having a D-List smile on her own 4-star ratings system, it's yours truly.

After all, I discovered my passion for dentistry after being transformed by my own dental experience back in high school. That's right; before I got my own A-List Smile I knew what it felt like to be insecure, even ostracized, because of my appearance.

Often the victim of jokes about my front teeth in both grade and middle school, I went to get braces at the age of 15. I was hopeful that by changing the way my teeth looked it would also change the way people felt about how I looked. But more importantly, I wanted it to change the way I felt about how I looked; and it worked! By the time I graduated high school I was voted "prettiest smile," completing a tremendous boost to my self-esteem.

The experience taught me a valuable lesson: words have meaning, and it's never okay when other people make fun of your appearance. I made a conscious decision to alter my appearance at a young age, and it has made all the difference in the world.

So I know firsthand the value of a brighter, straighter smile and the effects it can have on not just your smile, but your sense of self-esteem. That is why I created *5 Steps to a Hollywood A-List Smile*:

- **STEP 1:** *Assess Your Current Smile – A-List or D-List*
- **STEP 2:** *Learn the Benefits of an A-List Smile*
- **STEP 3:** *Prepare for Your A-List Smile*
- **STEP 4:** *Know What Products & Procedures Are On the Market, Which to Choose and Ways to Pay*
- **STEP 5:** *Care for Your A-List Smile*

By following these five steps closely, I will lead you through the minefield that is modern dentistry. Trust me, I know another boring book about this whitening procedure or that dental product is the last thing you're looking for in a book about A-List smiles; so what I've done is create a compelling and captivating, 5-step system that cuts to the chase.

I give you just what you need; no more, no less.

Dr. Catrise Austin with her favorite stars

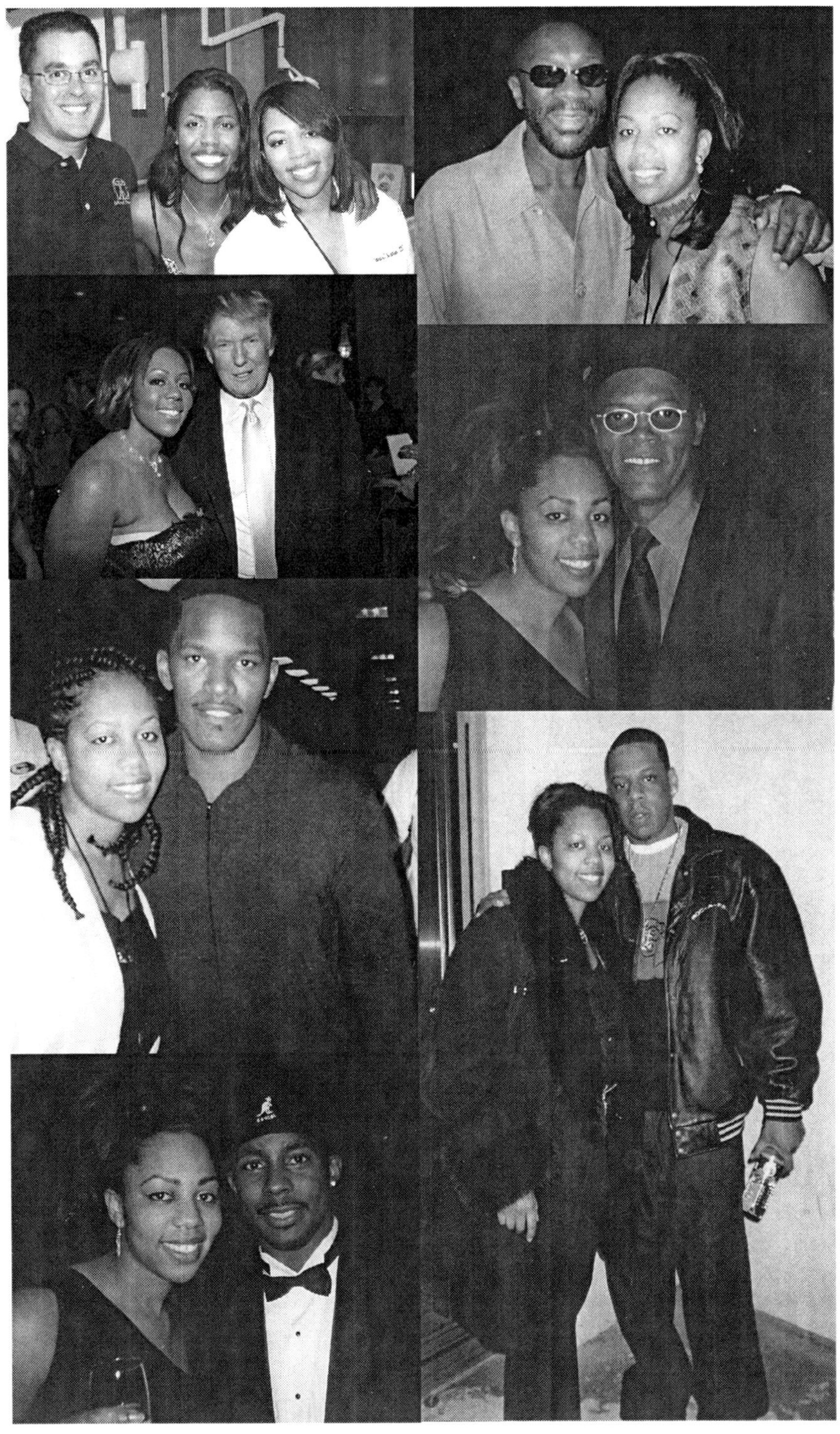

Dr. Catrise Austin with her favorite stars

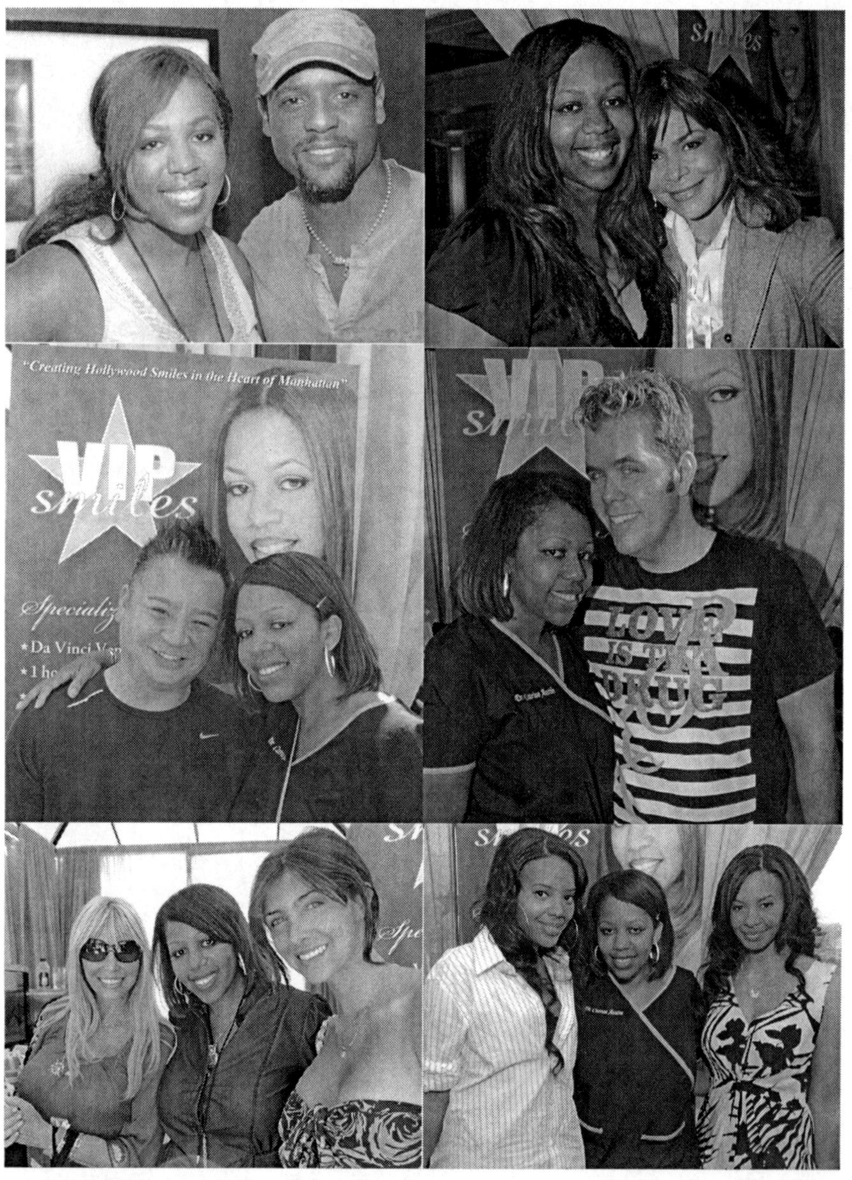

Introduction:

Give Your Smile the VIP Treatment

"Every time you smile at someone, it is an action of love, a gift to that person, a beautiful thing."

~ Mother Teresa

I did not come by my belief in having an A-List Smile by accident. They say that high school is a time when you discover what you'll do with the rest of your life; I guess you could say I bit off more than I could chew – in more ways than one.

As I began high school, I found myself being ashamed of opening my mouth. Not because I was a shy child by nature, but because of what my front teeth looked like. For years I'd been the butt of my classmates' jokes; all through grade and middle school to open my mouth at all meant to invite humiliation and rejection.

If you've ever been a victim of childhood cruelty, you'll know what I'm talking about; even if you haven't, you'll still know what I'm talking about. To be a child is to be insecure in the first place; to be a child with teeth that stand out for others to mock is to be insecure for a reason.

Neither is a very pleasant experience.

To keep from being laughed at or made fun of, I simply kept my smiles to a minimum. I became shy and reserved; a very different experience for a girl who'd grown up always seeing the glass as half-full. But such is the power of rejection; to endure it is to change yourself permanently.

Or maybe not so permanently.

I had always been a precocious child, maybe because I had been brought up to believe in myself – and that anything was possible. My mom had me when she was only seventeen, a teenager herself, and raised me as a single mom in none other than Flint, Michigan, then the 5th most dangerous city in the US!

Despite the challenges of raising a child on her own, or perhaps even because of them, my mom embraced motherhood as a teenager and took me everywhere she went. A lover of the arts, she took me to theater and to all of the concerts. I mean good ones, too, acts like Parlament/Funkadeliks, Rick James, even the Rick James VS Prince concert (when Prince first came onto the scene and nobody knew who he was—that's when I fell in love with him! At age 12).

I loved music; maybe because you could listen to it without seeing it. To someone self-conscious about her appearance, this was vitally important to me. The best part of all, I grew up in the beginning stages of hip hop, when Run DMC was new to the scene, then came the first hip hop tour; Fresh Fest (LL Cool J, Fat Boys, Whodini, UTFO, Run DMC) to which I was allowed to go.

My talent for meeting celebrities began back then at the age of 12. Run DMC came out with a song called "It's Like That." They came to little old Flint, MI, to a roller-skating rink. I was determined to meet them, so I wrote them a letter and slipped it under their dressing room door. Surprisingly, Russell Simmons (the unknown manager at the time) came out and said, "Who wrote this letter?"

I raised my hand and shouted, "Me, me!" He invited me and my friend into Run DMC's dressing room! The key thing is I got Russell's business card to "keep in touch." (By the way, I still have that card to this day.)

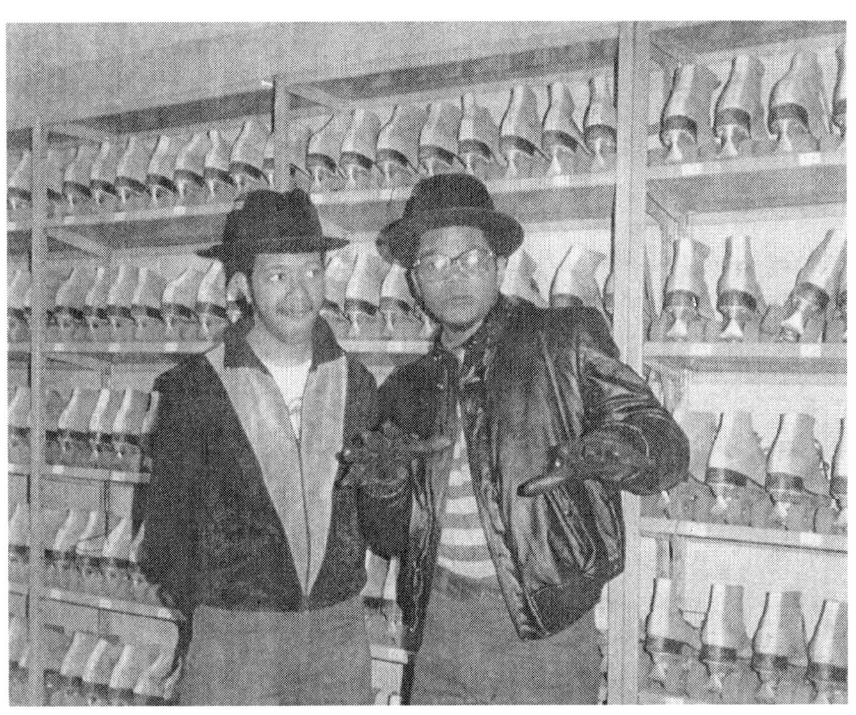

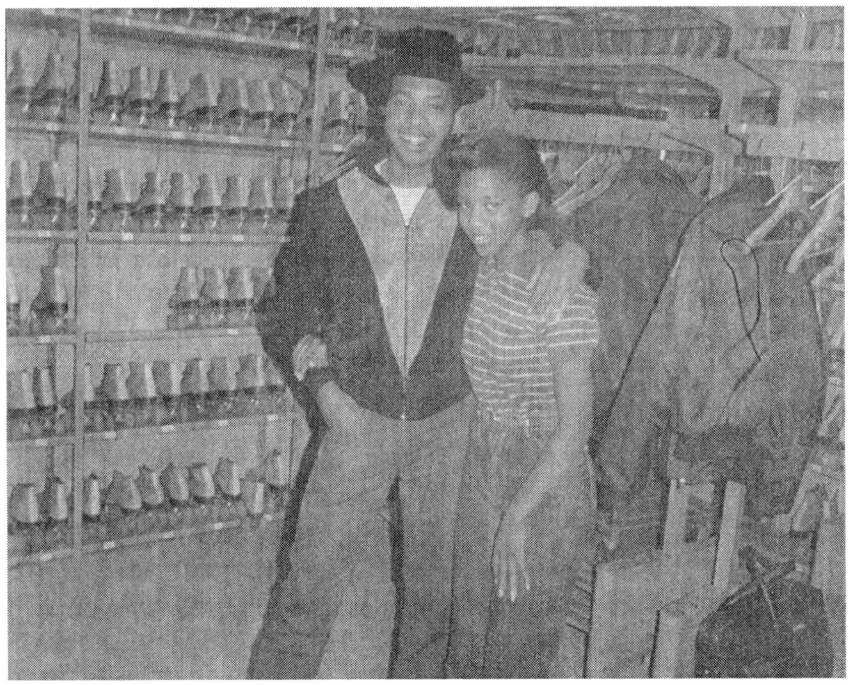

So a few months later the Fresh Fest Concert came to Saginaw, MI, it was in a big arena about the size of Madison Square Garden. In my head I thought, "Hey, I know Russell Simmons, so I'm going to go backstage and say 'Hello.' " Who did I think I was?

After the concert, I went to the security guard who was guarding backstage and I took out the business card of "my friend" Russell Simmons and said "I'm here to meet Russell Simmons – Run DMC's manager; see I have his card!"

Creative Music Promotions
Management - Promotion - Production
Kurtis Blow - Orange Krush - Jimmy Spicer
RUSH
1133 Broadway
N.Y., N.Y. 10010
Suite 404
President Russell Simmons (212) 620-0577

I flashed it to the guard and he said, "Oh, okay… come on back!" I couldn't believe that it worked! I didn't actually run into "my friend" this time, but I met and took pictures with the rap legends the Fat Boys and Whodini. That was huge for me at 12 years old, and one of the highlights of a period in my life where I didn't always have confidence. (Little did I know the art of meeting celebs would soon come in handy.)

I had noticed when I was younger that my teeth were different. There were spaces where there shouldn't be, noticeable ones; they just didn't come in like my friends' teeth. When you're in elementary school, you're prepared to be called "snaggle tooth" as you lose your baby teeth and get the big teeth. But my teeth were different and I knew it. (But when I look back at my young photos, I was always smiling.)

When did the smiling stop? When did those spaces in my teeth start to feel like a barrier between myself and the rest of the kids? I think when I started to develop into a "little woman" in middle school and high school; then I really started to feel a bit self-conscious about my looks, particularly my smile.

But what could I do? At that time, or so I thought, braces were out of the question. I knew that my mom didn't have the money to afford braces, so I was pretty much prepared to live with my imperfect smile. It wasn't until my family dentist asked me how I felt about my smile that I confided that I wasn't happy with it at all. Thank God, he shared my feelings with my mom. Knowing that my smile bothered me all my life and remembering how I'd been teased by kids (they called me "Bugs Bunny"), my mother decided to make the sacrifice.

And so at 15, I got braces! I was the first of my friends to get braces and everyone was happy for me. Even though they hurt like heck, I wore them proudly. At first I was self-conscious. I thought that maybe guys wouldn't like me as much with braces, but I still had IT! It took a month or so to get used to the food always getting stuck in my teeth! The good thing is that I became a teeth freak. I brushed more than ever because I never wanted to walk up to the cute guy in school, smile at him, and have an Egg McMuffin stuck in my teeth!

Even though I was wearing braces, I was still a nice looking young lady with a good personality. I knew that I only had to wear braces for a year, so each month was like a countdown for me. Each month you could see my spaces getting smaller and smaller and the transformation was encouraging.

The makeover was gradual, but striking; inch by inch, my front teeth weren't so prominent and gradually the rest of my mouth caught up with them. I was amazed; my whole face changed with the alignment, as did my attitude. While it took awhile for me to regain my natural sense of pride and self-esteem, by the time I graduated high school I was voted "prettiest smile."

The transformation was remarkable; in just a year I experienced a complete turnaround in how I viewed the world. Where before I was hesitant and timid, now I had confidence and hope. I didn't have to hold my hand over my mouth or smile without showing teeth, just to avoid embarrassment.

I could smile and laugh as big as I wanted – all because of how my teeth had changed. I realized then the power of a great smile; the power to heal and be healed, the power to overcome what had seemed like an insurmountable obstacle. My orthodontist had given me more than straighter teeth and a normal smile; he had literally given me my life back.

How did wearing braces and going from "Bugs Bunny" to "Prettiest Smile" change me? The monthly visits to the dentist and having to brush my teeth four times as much to keep them clean certainly made me more aware of teeth and dentistry overall. But it was the feeling of gratification and compliments that I received that boosted my self-esteem and made me want to become a dentist. I just wanted to provide that same life-changing experience to others.

My smile was a minor road block that, with the support of a caring mother and dentist, I was able to overcome. It taught me to be open and honest about the things that I needed to work on to improve myself. I learned that if you share your feelings and thoughts, just maybe someone will listen and help (even when you don't expect it) or at least present options of how to get help.

In my dental practice, I take the same approach that my dentist did with me. I always ask my patients what is on their dental "wish list" and what would they change about their smile if they could. I really listen to how they feel and look at their mannerisms as they share their feelings. It's the best feeling in the world to see someone literally change before your eyes after changing their smile.

It could be the smallest thing, from seeing someone happy with having the tartar and stains being removed from their teeth after a thorough cleaning or something big like seeing someone hold the mirror up to see their new smile makeover with porcelain veneers. Either way, the pleasure that I get is still the same. It's all about making my clients happy and I'm constantly reassured with feedback from my happy clients that I was born to be a dentist!

Looking back on it all, I cringe to think of how my future might have turned out had I not gotten braces when I did. How my senior year of high school would have been different; how my overall being would have been different. In fact, looking back I know that changing my appearance through dentistry helped me become a dentist in my own right.

In high school, I studied math and science. I was an all-A student, graduated with Honors and even won scholarships to fund my undergraduate studies. I attended the University of Michigan in Ann Arbor and maintained an above 3.0 GPA. My major was in psychology instead of science. I applied for Dental School and decided to move out of Michigan to Baltimore to attend the University of Maryland Dental School!

For the first time, I felt like I wasn't the smartest. The first two years of dental school were tough for me because I didn't have as much science background as my fellow classmates who had majored in science during their undergrad studies. My decision to study Psychology was biting me in the butt! The workload and information was a bit overwhelming for me and, for the first time, I was failing and didn't think that I could achieve this dream of mine; this burning goal to become a dentist.

In addition to my own insecurities, I had a boyfriend at the time, as well as classmates, who verbally expressed that they thought that I was "dumb" as a result of my periodic failures during my first two years of dental school. This really didn't help my self-esteem any. All I knew was that I had to get out of this academic slump and prove everyone wrong; prove that I was born to be a dentist!

But something changed during my third year. I started treating patients in the dental clinic and my light began to shine. I excelled in the dental clinic! I stayed late and came to clinic early to hone my skills. Whereas just a year earlier I had been an underachiever, now I became a superstar student, getting excellent grades and patients loved me!

I got my confidence back and I knew that I was going to make it to the finish line and win. I did so well that year that I finished my requirements early and was able to do specialty assignments that other students weren't privileged to do. In addition, my senior year presentation titled "HIV in Midlife and Elderly Patients," which was required for graduation, won several awards!

After eight years of college studies and finally reaching my goal, I decided to go and have some fun for a change in New York City, where I would be completing a year of hospital training in dentistry to get more experience.

That year not only did I hone my craft in my chosen profession but I had the time of my LIFE! New York was THE place to be in the late

'90s! Comedy clubs were packed, Hip Hop was in its golden years, and the dance clubs were unbelievable. Not to mention the opening of P. Diddy's new restaurant, Justin's. This was where, on any given Tuesday, you could run into celebrities like Mariah Carey, Busta Rhymes, Missy Elliot, New York Knicks players and, of course, P. Diddy himself!

Well, the light bulb began to burn bright in my head. Thinking about that young 12 year old girl that could work her way into concerts and meet celebs, I got an "ah ha" idea: I'm going to become the dentist to the stars in New York City!

What a crazy idea, right? I wasn't from New York City, I didn't know very many people, my family was back in Michigan and I had no support system in NY, and most importantly I HAD NO MONEY! Oh yeah, I was a young 28-year-old black woman in a man's world. Let's face it; dentistry is a field that is dominated by older, white men. Would people really support me as a dentist in The Big Apple? Could I REALLY get celebs to come to me?

11 years later… the answer is YES!!!!!!

Speaking of celebrities, I'll have you know that lots of famous TV, movie, music and hip-hop stars have had experiences just like mine. (And, I'm thinking, maybe a lot like yours as well.)

Rapper Kanye West used to get teased all the time in school about his appearance. As he writes in his autobiography, *Thank You and You're Welcome*, "My entire family used to tell me, 'You don't need to get your teeth fixed, they're fine,' but the kids in the lunchroom would say 'Your teeth are big and white just like a horse!'

"So I got braces and had to have eight teeth removed. Imagine [how] crowded my teeth must have been. After that I was teased for having braces. Once my teeth were fixed, everybody (including some of the same people who said I didn't need them) said, 'Your teeth look so much better!' So now, when I see people with messed-up teeth, I want to be that one person who tells them the truth like the kids told me, 'Your teeth are big and white like a horse!'"

Children can be cruel, but no crueler than a young girl might be to herself when staring back at a reflection that had caused her so much pain over the years. Learning to smile again was a rebirth of sorts – and I graduated with a new sense of confidence, strength and, most of all, a new sense of purpose.

Knowing that I wanted to become a dentist was a direct result of my own experience with a smile that had once shamed me. Now I wanted to give the gift of straighter, stronger, even whiter teeth to my own patients some day. I wanted to do for the world what my orthodontist did for me back when I was fifteen; give people their lives back with a new smile.

And so I come to you not just as another dentist writing another book on another new set of products and procedures; I come to you as a fellow sufferer from a not-so-A-List Smile. I know what it feels like to suffer from a lack of confidence so strong that it forces you not to smile, not to laugh, not to speak – even when it's your divine right to do so.

I could never write a book about improving your smile without including material about how it helps you be more confident, more trusting, more sincere and more hopeful about your own bright future.

Too often we think of going to the dentist as a mere chore that has to be done; this book will show that going to the dentist can be a real opportunity to find what's lacking in your own smile and give yourself the gift of an A-List Smile.

What, exactly, IS an A-List Smile? Well, that depends on you. One of our first orders of business will be to assess your current smile. Where is it, right now, on my 4-scale system? Is it A-List or D-List; C-List or B-List? Once we decide what's right for you, we can move on to discovering not just how to get an A-List Smile but also how to maintain it so that you never again have to feel anything other than confident about how you look – and how the world perceives you. Throughout this book I'll be talking about the latest and greatest in dental refinements, be they veneers or bonding, clear braces or bridges.

Below is a list of the dental products I will be detailing later on:

- **Porcelain Veneers**
- **Invisalign® Clear Braces**
- **ZOOM!® Teeth Whitening**
- **Snap-On Smile®**

- **Dental Bonding**
- **Tooth-Colored Fillings**
- **Dental Implants**

We'll weigh the costs associated with each procedure against the time constraints involved. I know you lead a busy, active, cost-conscious life so I'm here to guide you on how to get your A-List Smile within your financial budget and timeline.

You may not realize what's on the market today, which products really work and which don't. You may not understand the costs involved, the work that has to be done, how long a procedure might take or even how long it might take to heal between procedures requiring several visits. That's where I come in. My "starring role" as a celebrity dentist in the celebrity capital of the world – New York City – keeps me on the cutting edge of all the high-tech, latest products and procedures on the market today.

With an A-List Smile your life is vastly improved; not just physically, by brighter, straighter teeth but mentally as well, through a stronger sense of pride and self-confidence. At this point you may be asking yourself, "Hey, why is this dentist acting like my psychologist?"

My answer is simple; remember, I'm a little bit of both.

So don't consider this a book written by a dentist; read it like a book written by a friend. I do care about more than just your teeth; I care about your smile, and as I always say, "Your smile is the gateway to your personality; why close it off by feeling insecure or uncertain about it? Open it for the whole world to see!"

The quickest way to do just that is with an A-List Smile…

> *"Teeth are everything! It's the first thing that people notice about you. As a matter of fact, I pay really close attention to people's teeth."*
> **~ Jennifer Hudson**

Step 1:

Assess Your Current Smile – A-List or D-List

"All the statistics in the world can't measure the warmth of a smile."

~ Chris Hart

You know that feeling you get when a really hot new movie comes out? Sometimes the movie trailer makes the hairs on the back of your arms stand up on end or your friends can't stop talking about it or maybe the movie poster just makes your jaw drop or you read the book and loved it or your favorite star is in it. Whatever the reason, some movies are just meant to be on the A-List – others head straight to the bottom of the D-List.

Why is that? Why do some movies pop hot and others fall flat – like cold lead? Hollywood has been trying to figure it out for years, so if you think you're going to find the answer in a book written by a dentist, you're sadly mistaken. What I do know is that the recipe for every movie is pretty much the same: story, characters, plot, action, climax. So why doesn't every movie perform the same each weekend?

Well, lots of variables go into making a movie. Some stories are more interesting than others; some characters are more intriguing. Maybe this climax was more climactic while that one was anticlimactic;

maybe the two actors playing these intriguing characters just didn't have any chemistry. For whatever reason, even though all the same major elements are in every movie, not all movies are created equal.

Smiles are a lot like that. Just like every movie contains the basics of story, plot, character and action, every smile has the same basic elements: teeth, lips, gum, tongue and mouth. Look in a mirror right now and you'll see all five parties present and accounted for.

Don't stop there; walk around your office complex, neighborhood, shopping mall or bookstore and you'll see that everybody you encounter has the same basic tools to build an A-List Smile: teeth, lips, gum, tongue and mouth.

And yet, just like movies, not all smiles are created equal. Some smiles pop, bedazzle, thrill and energize; these are the A-List smiles, guaranteed to impress people at first glance. Other smiles are clean and bright but less than memorable; these are the B-List Smiles, good enough to pass muster under general inspection but not quite A-List or award-winning.

Some smiles are bland enough to be forgettable; we call these the C-List Smiles – not quite "best in show" but at least not last on our list, either. And, finally, there are those smiles that are memorable for all the wrong reasons; D-List Smiles that cry out for attention – *dental attention.*

Few people know what, exactly, makes the difference between an A-List Smile and one destined to go straight to the bottom of the D-List. You might say "crooked teeth" or "discoloration" or "red gums" or perhaps "an uneven mouth" might detract from your smile's A-List status, but you'd be wrong, technically speaking.

Check out any gossip mag or movie poster closely and you'll see that many of today's "hottest" A-List stars don't have the whitest or, for that matter, even the straightest teeth. Many stars, celebrities and even supermodels – if you broke their smile down, facet by facet – have less than perfect mouths but positively dazzling A-List smiles when the whole package comes together, with or without makeup. Likewise, someone with straight, white teeth, healthy gums and a perfectly symmetrical mouth can still have a D-List Smile – IF they haven't uncovered the secret to getting on the A-List.

Why is that? Well, as we've already learned, confidence has A LOT to do with how your smile is perceived. After all, what's the good of straight, white teeth if you're not confident enough to share them with the world?

Confidence plays a big part in any career, but particularly in the field of entertainment. Just ask rapper and movie star Common, who wore braces to correct some crooked teeth. "When I was young my bottom teeth were a little crooked and I got braces for both the top and the bottom," says the star of hit movies like *Street Kings* and *Wanted.* "Unfortunately, I wasn't too into the braces and I didn't go regularly to get them tightened. Eventually, I decided to let my friend take my braces off with his pliers. Hence in my young adult life I stood there with crooked teething wishing for straight ones."

Common discovered what so many of my patients do: don't try this at home! Eventually, he recognized the value of proper dental hygiene to his burgeoning music and movie career. "I started going to the dentist regularly because I always wanted to have a healthy set of teeth," he explains. "I was scared to get cavities because I had so many when I was a kid. For a while as an adult I would tell myself, 'I'm going to keep my teeth the way they are... a little crooked. That's natural.' Then at one point I saw my smile on the big screen and felt like I wanted it to be better."

As Common and so many of my other patients know, teeth and gums aren't all that go into an A-List Smile; how often you smile, how broadly, how genuine your smile is, its warmth and sincerity – these are all critical factors in getting, and keeping, an A-List Smile.

In this chapter I'll help you perform four critical tasks:

1.) Face Your Smile

2.) Quiz Your Smile

3.) Rate Your Smile

4.) Test Your Smile

All four are equally important; none can be done out of order. First, it's important to face your smile, own up to what you've got. Next you have to rate your smile, personally. How do YOU feel about it? We will quiz you on various aspects of your smile to see how your smile rates on our 4-star scale.

But it's just as important to test your smile out there, in the real world or, at the very least, for your friends and family during a private audience. How do THEY feel about your smile? Does it match how you, yourself, rated your own smile? Finally, after rating and testing your smile, if it's not exactly what you want you've got a whole book in which to find what's missing – and get it.

A-List Advice:

Few people know what, exactly, makes the difference between an A-List Smile and one destined to go straight on the D-List. Don't be afraid to face your smile; this task can change your life!

Face Your Smile:

The Mirror Test

If this suddenly feels like it will be a whole lot of work, relax; you're not alone. Many of my patients are surprised at how much work is involved in making the decision to alter their smile. But I don't want anyone making hasty decisions; it's important to really come face-to-face with your specific needs and how they relate to what might work – or not work – for you.

The first test is the ultimate challenge (for some): facing a mirror. Now it's time to see for ourselves what, exactly, your smile looks like; this way you can begin to rate it more accurately and be better prepared to face the rest of the book.

Here are the five steps to The Mirror Test:

1.) **Look in the mirror:** Seems like a no-brainer, sure, but have you ever *really* looked into the mirror? Sure, we glance at it from time to time throughout the day, usually as we pass by, but it's the rare person indeed who actually looks deep into the mirror and sticks around for what comes next. Even when we comb our hair or apply our makeup or fix our ties, we are often merely spot-checking a very specific area of our head, face or neck; we don't really soak in the whole picture. So the first step of The Mirror Test is to stand in front of a well-lighted mirror and look, really look, at yourself.

2.) **Smile**: Okay, now look at yourself and – smile. That's it; just smile. Smile like you normally would; not too wide, not too thin. Smile like you mean it, hold it and look at it. That's all; just smile.

3.) **Close your eyes**: Now close your eyes; that's right – smile and then close your eyes. Think about what you just saw; think about your smile. Think about the smile itself, then your face, then your head, then all of you. Think about how your smile worked individually, in a vacuum, and then think about how it looked as an accessory or part of the whole package.

4.) **Smile again**: Now open your eyes and smile again. Repeat Step 2, from above, and this time really, really concentrate on not just how your smile looks but how it makes you feel. Check your gut reaction to tell whether you are pleased, disappointed, shocked, relieved – or a combination of all four.

5.) **Write down your first impression:** Be quick, be bold, be brave and, most of all, be HONEST. The last step of The Mirror Test is to write down exactly which of the four smile ratings you feel like you qualify for, quickly, instantly, upon looking away from the mirror: A-List, B-List, C-List or D-List.

____

____

____

____

The "Rate Your Smile" Quiz

Let's face it; in our beauty-conscious society, one of the first things people notice about you is your smile. Now more than ever, with an economy spiraling downward and increased competition at work, a healthy, confident smile can be your calling card to success. You will see throughout this book how a strong, confident smile implies much more than personal hygiene; it truly radiates accomplishment, happiness, strength and success. All of these vital ingredients go to make a more successful, hardworking employee in the corporate workforce.

And let's say work isn't really your main focus when it comes to these sweeping changes when it comes to your appearance. What about romance? We all know it takes a lot of confidence to feel truly ourselves with someone we care about or, for that matter, to approach someone we're attracted to from afar. A healthy, brighter, whiter smile can give you the confidence you need to truly feel good about yourself. And who isn't attracted to a confident person?

So the next step on the road to that famous A-List Smile is to gauge your current smile using the "**Hollywood Smile Quiz" below.**

Take the Hollywood Smile Quiz

1. When you watch popular shows like *Americas Next Top Model* or *Project Runway*, what attracts you to the models' smiles?

____

____

____

____

____

____

2. Leading Actress Halle Berry is known for a confident, white, beautiful smile. How confident are you about your smile? On a scale of 1 through 10

Totally Unconfident **1--------------5--------------10** Very confident

What would you change?

____

____

____

____

____

____

3. Actor Tom Cruise is known for his distinct and uninhibited laughter. Do you hide or cover your smile when you laugh? If so, why?

____

____

____

____

____

____

4. Rap Legend DJ Biz Markie is not only famous for making music with his mouth but is also recognized by his gummy smile and small teeth. The appearance of your gums can play a huge role in the overall appearance of your smile. How do you rate your gums? Are they even in height and well proportioned to your smile? What color are your gums: pink or red?

____

____

____

____

____

____

5. For years, comedian Chris Rock never thought twice about the shape, size or position of his teeth. He admitted to Oprah Winfrey that when he finally realized that his teeth were not perfect, he immediately got veneers. How are your teeth shaped (too long, too short, too wide, too narrow)? Are your teeth misaligned?

____

____

____

____

____

____

6. Clients frequently ask me if they should close their gaps/spaces between their teeth, but superstar Madonna's trademark gap has been considered to be one of her sexiest traits. Do you have spaces? If so, how do you feel about them?

____

____

____

____

____

____

7. Earlier in his career, rapper Nas was known for having a chipped front tooth. He later went on to repair this imperfection and now has a beautiful smile. Are there any chips in your teeth? Are they uneven at the biting edges due to grinding?

____

____

____

____

____

____

8. Celebs like Julia Roberts and Mathew McConaughey are consistently named by the American Academy of Cosmetic Dentistry as having the "most beautiful smiles" in Hollywood. Not only are their teeth beautiful, but they appear to be clean and cavity free. How clean are your teeth? Any signs of plaque, tartar or coffee/tea stain? Any signs of cavities?

____

____

____

____

____

____

9. According to a foxnews.com report, several of Hollywood's leading men may not heat up the box offices if audiences could get a sniff of their bad breath! Having an A-List Smile means nothing if no one wants to get close to it because of halitosis. How confident are you about your breath? Do you have habits that contribute to bad breath? Do you constantly mask your breath with breath mints?

10. Next to teeth whitening and veneers, many celebs are flocking to remove unsightly silver fillings that often show on screen and in photos. Do you have silver fillings that are visible in your smile? Does the silver appearance bother you?

Use My Hollywood Ratings System

Hollywood is a place where everybody wants to be ranked somewhere, from the Best-Dressed List to World's Sexiest to Most Powerful Player. But what if you could rate your smile? Now you can with my simple Hollywood Ratings System:

1. **The "A-List" Smile (4 Stars – ****):** People with A-List smiles know it – and are not afraid to share with the world how confident and beautiful they feel. It's the smile worthy of the red carpet; the A-List Smile we're all shooting for when we wake up in the morning and pay such close attention to our appearance. This smile is marked by a wide range of positive characteristics, including:

    - **No visible cavities or fillings**
    - **Clean teeth (no evidence of plaque or tartar)**
    - **Straight teeth**
    - **Teeth in proportion to your mouth (not too big or too small; not too short or too long)**
    - **Healthy gums (pink in color)**
    - **White teeth with lack of discoloration (yellow, brown, gray or black)**
    - **Fresh, pleasant breath accompanied by confidence**
    - **Even, uniform and proportioned gum line and not "too gummy"**

2. **The "B-List" Smile (3 Stars – ***):** The B-List Smile has the same basic characteristics as the A-List Smile, only certain changes are developing to help it lose some of its natural luster and shape. These include:

    - **Moderately clean teeth (slightly visible evidence of bacterial plaque or tartar)**

- **Mild yellowing (or other discoloration of teeth, such as brown, gray or black)**
- **Mild rotations, spaces or other misalignments**
- **Hesitance or reluctance to smile**
- **Minor flaws (chips; worn enamel)**
- **No visible cavities or fillings**
- **A semi-confident smile**
- **Fresh, pleasant breath**

3. **The "C-List" Smile (2 Stars – **):** Signs of the C-List Smile include:

    - **Visible cavities (brown or black spots/discolorations)**
    - **Visible old fillings or crowns (old silver fillings or old bondings becoming noticeable)**
    - **Moderate buildup of plaque and tartar that is visible when you smile**
    - **Moderate yellowing or other discolorations (brown, grey or black)**
    - **Moderate flaws in alignments (moderately crooked; moderate spacing or gaps)**
    - **More noticeable flaws (sizable chips, moderately worn enamel)**
    - **Red, swollen gums**
    - **An uneven gum line (or a "gummy" smile)**

4. **The "D-List" Smile (1 Star – *):** Here are the indicators of a D-List Smile:

    - **Obvious neglect due to infrequent dental visits, accompanied by very little to no smiling**
    - **Large, noticeable cavities**

- **Visible old fillings or crowns**
- **Severe tartar buildup that is noticeably visible**
- **Severe yellowing or other discoloration**
- **Severe flaws in alignment**
- **Red, swollen gums**
- **Loose teeth**
- **Uneven gum line**
- **Accompanied by bad breath from lack of dental care**

The beauty of my 4-star rating system is that, just like an A-List Smile, it depends on who's doing the rating. My job is to help you understand the pros and cons of each type of smile – and what can be done to rectify your current smile **<u>if you so desire</u>**.

Remember, smiling is about a lot more than teeth and gums; how you *think* you look plays a big part in how you rate your smile – and how you rate your smile has a lot to do with how often, and how wide, you smile.

As you can see, the A-List Smile is perfect. Meanwhile, each smile has its own unique properties that help to give it a higher, or lower, ranking on my 4-Star scale. The good part about this chapter is that it's written just for YOU; no one has to know you ever took this test or, for that matter, what kind of smile you had at the very beginning of this process.

The beauty of change is that it's an evolution; none of my products, procedures, techniques or tips changes you overnight. Even if it's an "instant" procedure like teeth-whitening, the true change occurs over time as you truly begin to embrace and share your brighter, white teeth with the world at large.

Take this chapter, and this time, seriously; embrace this period in your life where you are about to embark on change and prepare yourself, mentally and physically, for the A-List Smile that awaits.

Remember that change is a process; there is no deadline or "expiration date" for any decision you make as a result of reading this book. These quizzes, tests and questionnaires are designed to help you get to know yourself better so you can be fully prepared to make the right decision for you – at the right time for you.

Test Your Smile:

From 4-Star to 1-Star

So, how did you do? A-List, B-List, C-List or D-List Smile? Didn't rate yourself? Go back and do it! Don't worry; I'll wait. I'm serious here, because this is very serious business. To know what you want to do with your smile you need to know how to rate your smile – and what rating it deserves.

Or maybe you rated yourself and came up short of your expectations. Don't worry; there's a light at the end of the tunnel. A smile is something many of us think about only when necessary – like those twice-yearly reminders we get from our friendly dentist's office. But something made you buy a book called *5 Steps to a Hollywood A-List Smile*, be it a nagging doubt from your childhood that your smile wasn't all it could be or a recent comment from someone you know and trust – or even a complete stranger – so I want you to get your money's worth. That's why our next step is to test your smile, and that means making a "test run" in front of some very special people.

The Audience Response:

Talking with Family, Friends, Coworkers and/or Classmates

Can you trust yourself to accurately rate your smile? Might you be rating it *too* harshly, putting yourself in the D-List category when you're actually more of a B-List Smile? Or maybe you're seeing your smile through rose-colored glasses and think you've got an A-List Smile when others might peg you as a C-List – or worse?

That is why I urge you to "test your smile" – out in the real world – by asking others to rate it as well. I think you'll agree that the following people can be very useful in helping you see yourself – and your smile – a LOT more clearly:

- **Family:** If there is one group of people you should be able to trust to tell it to you straight, it should be your family. Let them know your concerns about your current smile (they may already know), either one-on-one or as a small group, and speak to them openly, honestly and sincerely about your hopes, concerns, dreams and fears. Don't forget that genetics play a large part of how your mouth – including your teeth and gums – were formed. Ever heard someone tell a baby, "She has her mother's (or father's) smile?" That's genetics; take a look around the room as you talk to your family and rate their smiles; while you're at it, rate each other's. Discuss what you like and dislike about your smiles and, chances are, by the time you've passed the "family test" you will feel a whole lot better about your smile – no matter how you rated it yourself.

- **Friends:** Your friends can be an invaluable source of comfort and support when it comes to rating, then testing, your smile. Unlike family, with whom you share a different dynamic, I recommend testing your smile on friends during a one-on-one basis. Pick a casual setting and ask them to "rate" your smile; they don't need to know the Hollywood ratings system we use – 1 to 4 stars should work just fine. When they're done, tell them WHY they're rating your smile and see if the rating changes. Ask them to be open and honest; don't be afraid of what they may have to say and trust their friendship to guide them to be as straightforward and candid as possible.
- **Coworkers and/or Classmates:** I've combined the next two test groups – coworkers and/or classmates – into one group because they're different than the first two groups. In other words, they don't have the emotional attachment to you that family and friends do, so you can't always trust them to be perfectly honest. But what I really want you to do is to casually gauge how your coworkers and/or classmates respond to your smile. (If you're lucky, you may get an honest response as to how they feel about your smile.) If you're someone who doesn't often smile, start smiling more often and be mindful of the responses you get. Do people smile back without seeming to know why? Do people automatically look down at your smile and nod favorably – or cringe noticeably? With this particular group, you're looking for visual clues versus verbal clues; it's not what they say so much as how they look when they see you smile. Or maybe you're someone who smiles often but just as often takes smiling for granted, assuming that everyone is smiling back because of your warmth and sincerity. For the next few days pay attention to how people react to your smile; their faces, eyes and expressions may be telling you volumes!

A-List Advice:

Discuss what you like and dislike about your smile and, chances are, by the time you've passed the "family test" you will feel a whole lot better about your smile – no matter how you rated it.

A Picture's Worth a Thousand Words:

Perusing Old Photographs

Some of us are born with A-List smiles but gradually let them fade to B-List, then C-List Smiles until, finally, you wind up with a D-List Smile – and don't know why.

Some of us suspect we might know why our smiles aren't exactly A-List at the moment, but don't quite realize how our bad habits can contribute to less-than-A-List smiles. For instance, smoking isn't the only bad habit that can turn an A-List Smile into a frown; heavy coffee and tea drinkers can also lend a hand in discoloring their teeth.

Sugar, chocolate, soda and other junk foods can help deteriorate precious tooth enamel, and even just such little ticks as chewing ice or sucking on lemons can help contribute to a less-than-stellar smile. Here are 16 of the most frequent contributors to poor oral health and a D-List Smile:

1. Poor oral hygiene habits such as improper brushing and flossing techniques
2. Infrequent dental visits for checkups and maintenance
3. Genetic/family history of gum disease
4. Medical health conditions such as diabetes, HIV/AIDS and even pregnancy can affect your ability to heal from gum disease

5. Poor diet/nutrition
6. Long-term intake of certain medications (like tetracycline) can affect the color of your smile
7. Stress can cause people to develop grinding and teeth clenching behaviors, which lead to chips and worn enamel
8. Poor brushing and flossing techniques, such as using a hard- or medium-bristled toothbrush, can remove enamel at the gum line and/or cause the gums to move up the tooth, causing root exposure or notches in the teeth. Not flossing properly can still leave hidden plaque below the gums, causing gum disease to form
9. Misuse of your teeth, such as using them to open bottles, chewing ice, chewing on bones, chewing pencils or pens or eating extremely hard foods or candy
10. Not immediately replacing teeth that have been pulled causes your teeth to shift and lean
11. Not wearing a retainer to maintain your smile after your parents paid for braces!
12. Daily consumption of foods and beverages that can stain your teeth (i.e. coffee, tea, dark berries and red wine, etc.)
13. Daily habits such as smoking can stain your teeth and ruin the color of your smile
14. Tongue rings are known to commonly hit the upper teeth and cause minor chips and major fractures
15. Eating disorders such as bulimia can erode the tooth's enamel
16. Exposing your teeth without a mouth guard during contact or extreme sports can put your smile at risk.

The good news is that every factor on the above list is reversible; we can help each other find a way to that coveted A-List Smile. In fact, did you know there is a handy little tool up in your attic or hiding in your closet that can give you an accurate timeline of just how your smile has looked over the decades? That's right; it's called the family photo album and this is your next step to getting an A-List Smile: perusing old photographs for a reminder as to how your smile has evolved.

Take it out now and start at the very beginning – with your baby pictures. Follow your development from childhood through the teen years, then college and beyond, up until your most recent photographs. Don't have any recent ones? That could be pretty telling evidence; people who don't like their smiles often avoid or downright refuse to have their pictures taken.

If you are a born ham and have plenty of current photos, examine them closely to see how they stack up to your more youthful snapshots. Has your smile gotten better over time, or worse? Is what you're seeing in all those side-by-side photo comparisons matching up with your own smile self-rating and what your family, friends, coworkers and/or classmates told you?

My patients find this to be a very useful exercise when I give them their "Photo Album Homework." Again, we're talking about change – this time for the good – and cultivating healthy habits to reinforce the change. Seeing how your smile, and even your overall appearance, has changed over time can help you stop making bad decisions and start making good ones again. And don't worry; no one will ever grade you – other than yourself, that is. What you're looking for here, of course, is threefold:

1.) Visual evidence of what kind of smile you had

2.) How it's evolved over the years

3.) And, finally, what it looks like today

Think of these aspects of your smile as guideposts revealing changes that may have occurred in the evolution of your smile. By focusing on these three factors you can get a clearer picture of what your smile looks like now versus then.

A-List Advice:

Did you know there is a handy little tool up in your attic or hiding in your closet that can give you an accurate timeline of just how your smile has looked over the ages? That's right; it's called the family photo album. Take it out now; this is your next step to getting an A-List Smile.

Great Expectations:

Knowing What You Want Out of Your Smile

Shawn Kirkaldy grew up in Brooklyn, New York. Today he is a Physical Education teacher for Pre K-8th grades at a Catholic school in Harlem. Shawn considers himself a "happy camper," but he didn't always have a reason to smile. When he was a child, Shawn recalls, "I remember my smile was shattered when my brother tripped me in the street and I fell face first to the pavement and broke one of my two front teeth."

Despite this D-List setback, Shawn continued to have an A-List outlook on life. "The majority of my photos [growing up] capture me smiling. I never knew how *not* to smile, and my mom smiled a lot, too. [I guess] I'm always smiling because I love life and God sent friends I share this journey with."

For many years, Shawn took his chipped tooth in stride. "I never felt I needed to be ashamed or otherwise because of my chipped tooth when I was young," he admits. But things started to change for Shawn when he got a little older. "I wished I had a nicer smile when I became a young adult while working for the NBA as an intern."

Like many of my patients, Shawn had a very specific reason for feeling insecure about his smile and wanting to get it off the D-List. "I wanted to meet and date a more mature and polished lady," he confessed.

I met Shawn recently and was able to take his smile from D-List to A-List with some very simple procedures. Afterward, Shawn was surprised by "…the fact that my new teeth looked so natural and real!" Shawn and I were both satisfied that his smile was red carpet worthy.

More importantly, however, Shawn gained a new sense of confidence in himself that he didn't even realize he was lacking. "What a life-altering experience," he says of the first time he looked in the mirror after getting his A-List Smile. "What a confidence booster to smile ever the more and the feeling that I had arrived fully as an adult. I felt like I was a rock star! I felt I could meet and greet any person and 'Wow' them with my smile and I did – and still do!"

How does Sean feel today? He says, "I feel blessed that my dentist, yes, my dentist single-handedly raised my level of acceptance in life and the overwhelming gravitation of the opposite sex."

What were the two biggest things Shawn's A-List Smile has done for him? "The most important thing my new smile has done for me," says Shawn, "is that my children and family members now realize the wonder [of] what a rock star smile does for an individual in the professional and personal area of his/her life. My smile often conjures the thought that I've lived a higher status life, since having good teeth and a smile is often synonymous with success and wealth.

"The second most important thing my smile has done for me is that it creates conversation and compliments that come at a rapid pace. The first thing women and men alike say to me is, 'Wow, you have a great smile!' With me being relatively young in age, having such a great smile is believed to [be] natural and not cosmetic, and my teeth look, feel and shine like natural teeth."

Finally, Shawn has an inspiring message to share with people who aren't happy with their smile: "I tell all of my friends, relatives and coworkers if they aren't happy with their smile, for a relatively small investment (no investment is too great if it enhances your life as having great teeth do) you can be just like me, with a rock star smile. Also, that they may go through some slight discomfort and mild pain, but the rewards are 1,000% worth every bit of it. Having a beautiful smile is as important as obtaining a college degree; you may be able to live, work and survive without one, but when you have one, the confidence to achieve what you set out to achieve is boundless!"

Fortunately for you, you've already got a leg up on Shawn; this book didn't exist when he got his A-List Smile. (No wonder he was so surprised with his results!) But you? You've had over 50-pages of preparation and insight to help you form your own expectations for an A-List Smile.

So, now that you've rated your smile, tested your smile and actually faced your smile, it's time for a little downtime. Turn away from the mirror, let the previous sections of this chapter germinate and start to think bout what, exactly, it is that you want out of your smile – and the rest of this book.

Maybe you're a businessman who realizes his current smile is affecting sales (and not in a good way). Perhaps you're a student who sits in the back of the class and covers her face when she is called upon because you're so insecure about your smile. Maybe you're an actor or model who wants to complete your hip, suave look with that A-List Smile. Maybe you're a busy mom who simply needs a reason to smile.

Whatever your reasons for changing your smile, before we move on to Step 2, I want you to ask yourself the following two questions:

- **Is this just a cosmetic change – or a healthier change?** There is no "right" or "wrong" answer to this question, only a better understanding of why you're reading this book and what you hope to get out of it.
- **How far am I willing to go for change?** This is not some extreme adventure where you're going to be testing yourself to see how many products and procedures you can endure. You simply want to be aware, going forward, of your tolerance for things like multiple office visits, downtime while you recover, possible costs involved and/or how comfortable you are in the dentist's chair.

Knowing the answers to – or at least being aware of – these two questions now, as we move forward, will help you better understand and rate each product and procedure on your own personal scale of possibility.

A-List Advice:

Turn away from the mirror, make time for yourself, let the previous sections of this chapter germinate and start to think bout what, exactly, it is that you want out of your smile. If it helps, write it down and save it for later; see if you met your goals once you have your A-List Smile.

Reflections of a Smile

Okay, so there you have it. You've **tested**, **rated** and **faced** your smile. How did you do? Not that easy, huh? But there's a method to my madness; my patients tell me that without Step 1 of getting their A-List Smile, they might not have been prepared for what came next. I don't want the same to happen to you.

The best part of what we've just accomplished is that now you know what your smile really looks like, how you feel about it, what people say about it, how it looks and even how it feels to look at it; believe it or not, this is priceless information.

With this information you can change your world forever. Maybe you realized that it won't take that much to get that A-List Smile; maybe you came to the realization that it's going to be harder than you thought. Either way, you KNOW; and knowledge is power.

This power is going to help you in future chapters as I introduce the various products and procedures on the market today to help you get your A-List Smile. If the opposite is true, and a whitening treatment or two just won't cut it at this point, at least the first time you're hearing this won't be in the dentist chair; you already KNOW what it is you need.

A-List Advice:

Now you know what your smile really looks like, how you feel about it, what people say about it, how it looks and even how it feels to look at it; believe it or not, this is priceless information. With this information, you can change your world forever!

"A beautiful smile warms people up to you. It gives you confidence, especially in the entertainment industry."

~ Rhianna

Step 2:

Learn the Benefits of an A-List Smile

"Of all the things you wear, your expression is the most important."

~ Janet Lane

Dale Carnegie, author of the groundbreaking book *How to Win Friends and Influence People*, wrote, "The expression one wears on one's face is far more important than the clothes one wears on one's back."

Was he right? You be the judge. Take a look at your most successful business books and pay close attention to the author on the front cover. What is he or she doing? Smiling. Jack Welch on the cover of *Winning*? Smiling. Carolyn Kepcher on the cover of *Carolyn 101*? Smiling. Lee Iacocca on the cover of *Where Have All the Leaders Gone*? Smiling.

Coincidence? I think not. But how can something as simple as a smile help us to succeed in a world where smiles are so rare? A more important question might be how can *not* smiling hurt us professionally – or otherwise?

John Samuel, Success correspondent for AskMen.com explains, "The simple action of keeping your head up high and smiling when acknowledging someone conveys confidence and a demand for respect. It is pretty simple; if you show people that you are confident and friendly, they will be more responsive to you. This friendly environment will create a positive climate for trust and business."

Bill Brooks writes in *American Salesman*, "Smiling fosters a positive atmosphere, which is exactly what you want if you hope to eventually finalize any transaction." Finally, in his new book ***Walking Tall:*** *Key Steps to Total Image Impact*, personal branding consultant and author Lesley Everett explains, "A smile is a fundamental business tool and… one that is forgotten about most of the time, especially when we are nervous."

In these changing times, you'll need every leg-up you can have at work. A smile exudes confidence; confidence creates trust. Now more than ever your employers – or even employees – are looking for competent, capable, confident people who can find success even when it's getting harder and harder to come by; having a strong, confident smile gives you that leg up at work.

No matter what field you're in, dental hygiene is extremely important. Just ask boxer Maureen Shea, who was Hillary Swank's main sparring partner as the actress prepared for her Oscar-winning role in the movie, *Million Dollar Baby.* "I got braces in kindergarten, as a very small child, and after having them for seven years, my mouth and teeth were totally corrected," Maureen explains. "My parents were adamant about me having this done and now, as an adult, I am glad they insisted."

Now, thanks to straight teeth and a daily dose of dental hygiene, Maureen enjoys the confidence her A-List Smile gives her. "As a public figure I do a lot of speaking, and it's nice to be complimented and told I have a great smile and teeth. It boosts my confidence when speaking to the press, at a speaking engagement or just one-on-one with fight fans. That makes my dental regimen – brushing three times a day AND flossing – something I take seriously. I am also extremely conscious of keeping my teeth and smile protected in my sport. Being a professional boxer, you learn to protect yourself, and my mouth and teeth are no exception. I use a custom made mouth guard molded specifically for my teeth. This mouth guard protects my teeth, my gums, and my jaw, and also serves as a preventive measure for minor jaw and head injuries."

We've all heard the term "dress for success." There are even dozens of books to teach you *how* to dress for success, but as Manhattan's dentist to the stars I'm here to tell you that before anyone looks at your shoes, your watch, your blazer, your purse, your tie, your dress or even your resume – they look at your smile.

We all know this one basic fact to be true: when you look better, you feel better. And when you feel better, you do better; when you do better, you are a happier, healthier, more successful person. It may be possible to become an executive without The A-List Smile, but in today's world it's nearly impossible to be an *effective* executive without The A-List Smile.

By now we have determined what kind of smile you have, based on my four-star rating list. Be prepared for that to change, and here's why: no matter what you think your smile looks like now, there is always room for improvement.

Maybe you're not convinced that you need an A-List Smile; I understand. It's my business to give people the A-List Smile, so sometimes I take it for granted. In this chapter I will leave no doubt in your mind about the various health, physical, personal, emotional and spiritual benefits of an A-List Smile.

There is so much to recommend a healthier, brighter, whiter, stronger smile that I really felt you needed a whole step just to appreciate them all. Ready? Good, cause I really can't wait any longer to share them all with you:

A-List Advice:

We all know this one basic fact to be true: when you look better, you feel better. And when you feel better, you do better; when you do better, you are a happier, healthier, more successful person.

A Healthy Mouth is a Healthy Life

When it comes to proper dental hygiene, people always think dentists are strictly doctors who work on your mouth; technically, I suppose, this definition is accurate. But it doesn't quite do justice to how important a healthy smile is to a healthy life.

The truth is, good oral hygiene forms a barrier against diseases entering your body. In the past, researchers have linked gum disease such as gingivitis with an array of serious health concerns such as diabetes, stroke, premature birth and hypertension.

It might seem odd that the mouth could be the gateway to such broad-scope diseases, but think about that for a minute: everything you eat and drink goes through the mouth. You breathe, cough, swallow, talk and ingest through the mouth. It is, in effect, the point of entry for all of the body's nutrients – as well as many of its infections.

Writing on behalf of the *Herald & Review*, reporter Annie Getsinger says, "The relationship between good oral hygiene and a healthy body might not be immediately evident, but dentists say thorough, proper flossing, brushing and professional teeth cleaning can help those with chronic illnesses ward off infection."

And according to The American Academy of Periodontology, "Infections in the mouth can play havoc elsewhere in the body. Since July of 1998, evidence has continued to mount to support these links."

They add, "Periodontal bacteria can enter the blood stream and travel to major organs and begin new infections. Research is suggesting that this may:

- Contribute to the development of heart disease, the nation's leading cause of death.
- Increase the risk of stroke.
- Increase a woman's risk of having a preterm, low birth weight baby.
- Pose a serious threat to people whose health is compromised by diabetes, respiratory diseases, or osteoporosis." [Source: www.perio.org]

So, clearly, your smile is more than just teeth and gums; think of your mouth as a force field, or barrier, between yourself and bad health. Keeping your mouth, and thus your smile, healthy is your first step in a healthier, happier life.

It's important to remember that a smile is much more than appearance; having a "healthy" smile truly does have health benefits. In turn, those health benefits ripple and reverberate throughout every other area of your life. Looking good is great; feeling good is even better. The best part is, having an A-List Smile accomplishes both amazing feats!

A-List Advice:

Good oral hygiene forms a barrier against diseases entering your body.

Your (Many) Health Benefits, Courtesy of an A-List Smile

I believe strongly that the body and the mind are connected; I also believe that they are connected in just that order: first the body, then the mind. Don't get me wrong, your mind is the magical seat of all imagination, stimulation and creation that goes on in your life – but without the body there would be nothing to imagine, stimulate or create. So in this section we start out with how the smile affects your entire body; and boy, does it ever!

Sometimes getting your teeth bonded can mean the difference between a D-List and an A-List Smile; other times it means the difference between insecurity and confidence. Sherene Hudson grew up in Jamaica, Queens. Today, she's a Contract Coordinator in the Business & Legal Affairs department at a Media Entertainment Company. Growing up, Sherene smiled a lot but, she admits, "I was always aware of the spaces in my teeth."

Like most children unhappy with their smiles, Sherene swallowed her feelings and put on a brave face for the outside world. "I remember many photos of myself smiling," she says before confessing, "but I was smiling for the cameras."

Many of my patients don't become insecure about their smiles until early- to late-adolescence. For Sherene, things started much earlier. "My siblings used to tease me on a regular basis when I smiled in front of them; they were the first ones to make me a little insecure about my smile." How early did her insecurities start? "My being self-conscious started as a child around the age of 8 years old."

Later in life Sherene put behind her the voices of her family critics and, instead, became her own harshest critic. "As a young adult," she admits, "I was very much aware of the spaces in my teeth, but it didn't bother me as much; people would always tell me that I had a nice smile, but I wasn't satisfied with it."

It was then that she began thinking seriously about getting an A-List Smile. "I thought about a nicer smile from the age of 16 to an adult," she says. "I always pay attention to teeth and smiles, and when I would see people who had nice smiles, it really made a difference on how their face looked to me. I just feel like a nice smile exudes confidence."

What was the biggest part of Sherene's decision to change her smile? "I just wanted a beautiful smile," she says. "Closing the spaces in my teeth has been on my dental 'wish list' for over two years. I made a promise to myself that I would be improving my smile at the beginning of the year."

Once I had bonded Sherene's teeth, she said, "The most surprising part was the fact that my smile and face was changed in a matter of hours. After my bonding procedure, I was so happy; I just couldn't stop smiling when I got home."

Today Sherene is more than satisfied with her A-List Smile. "My teeth look and feel great," she told me recently. "It doesn't even feel like I had anything done. My teeth just look great!"

Sherene said she never feel insecure about her smile now that she's had bonding to remove the spaces in her teeth. "My new teeth have given me more confidence in myself as well as my smile," she says. "I just want to talk and smile all day. By making these improvements, I feel like I'm putting me first by making my outside become as beautiful as I am on the inside."

Not surprisingly, Sherene has some parting words for anyone considering who isn't happy with their smile: "I tell all of my friends that they have options and to go see Dr. Austin."

What are the specific health benefits of smiling? After reading this section, I think you may be asking yourself, "What AREN'T the health benefits of smiling?" That's because there are so many! Here are a few surprising ones that will make you want to smile more:

- **Smiling is a natural pain killer:** According to Mark Stibich, Ph.D., of About.com, "Smiling is a natural drug." How? Says Dr. Stibich, "Studies have shown that smiling releases endorphins, natural pain killers, and serotonin. Together these three make us feel good."
- **Three more health benefits:** Dr. Stibich also claims that smiling can relieve stress, boost your immune system and even lower your blood pressure.
- **Be more optimistic, positive and motivated:** Says psychologist Dr. David Lewis, "Seeing a smile creates what is termed as a 'halo' effect, helping us to remember other happy events more vividly, feel more optimistic, more positive and more motivated."
- **Just like chocolate:** According to The British Dental Health Foundation, "…a smile gives the same level of stimulation as eating 2,000 chocolate bars. The results were found after scientists measured brain and heart activity in volunteers as they were shown pictures of smiling people and given money and chocolate."
- **Can your yearbook picture and, more specifically, whether you were smiling predict your future?** Two researchers claim that, yes, it can. Writing in the *Journal of Personality and Social Psychology*, researchers and authors LeeAnne Harker, PhD, and Dacher Keltner, PhD, of the University of California, Berkeley, said, "Over time, women who expressed more positive emotion in their yearbook pictures became more organized, mentally focused and achievement-oriented, and less susceptible to repeated and prolonged experiences of negative affect."

I could go on and on like this all day (just ask my patients!), but I think you get the picture by now; smiling doesn't just make you happier, it actually makes you physically and mentally healthier!

A-List Advice:

A smile gives the same level of stimulation as eating 2,000 chocolate bars.

It's Impossible to Be Insecure When You're Smiling

Aside from the various health issues we've discussed in this section (and don't they make you feel even better about smiling?!?), your smile can protect you from something just as debilitating as high blood pressure or an infection: insecurity.

Ebony grew up in Shreveport, Louisiana. Today she is an aspiring model who plans on getting into acting. Obviously, for someone wanting a red carpet career, getting an A-List Smile is practically a mandatory job requirement.

Growing up, Ebony remembers "... how small my teeth were and I was always smiling. Smiling was second nature to me," she remembers, "behind dancing. I was usually smiling in pictures when I was with people I love, someone said something funny, or I was striking a pose."

Like many children, Ebony enjoyed a carefree youth full of free, easy smiles. "I didn't really become self-conscious about my smile," she remembers, "until I was a teenager. That's when my smile started to bother me."

By then Ebony had entered the world of beauty pageants and suddenly found herself being compared to others; and comparing herself to others. Insecurity quickly followed. "I was in high school," she recalls. "I was doing pageants and all the other girls had perfect teeth and, while I liked my smile, I felt it could've been better."

Already an experienced beauty pageant winner, Ebony later decided she wanted to pursue modeling and acting as a career; that's when her concerns about her smile went from D-List to A-List. "I really wanted to change it for my career and for self-confidence," she recalls.

After getting a Snap-On Smile, Ebony was pleased with the results and "how quick the procedure was."

"I was so relieved," she adds, "and emotional. It was like looking at a completely different person!"

Months later Ebony is still beaming about her A-List Smile. "I don't even think about it [anymore]; it feels so natural." But beyond her appearance, Ebony is happy she had the procedure for several equally important reasons. "It's relieved a lot of stress," she explains. "It's given me confidence and renewed my love of smiling!"

What would Ebony tell someone who isn't happy with their smile? "Don't think about it," she warns. "It's so important to get it fixed as soon as possible. You really do feel like a new person inside and out!!"

Many of us struggle with insecurity in both our personal and professional lives; this fact becomes even more magnified when we are actually insecure **because of our smiles**. Take an already insecure person and double that insecurity because of crooked, misshapen or discolored teeth and he or she becomes a veritable "insecurity factory."

But there is hope for these people; there is hope for you. By being prouder of your smile you become less insecure. In fact, regardless of how your smile looks right now, I have found that it is impossible to feel insecure when you are smiling.

Don't believe me? Try it for yourself. I try this experiment with my insecure patients all the time and they are amazed by how a simple thing like smiling can literally boost their ego – and do away with their insecurity. At least, temporarily.

According to June M. Lay M.S., founder and director of The Nutrition Center located in New York City, "Social psychology research bears out that facial expressions do reflect our inner feelings, and changing our facial expression can help to change our feelings, too. The results of studies show that different facial expressions are accompanied by changes in physiological activity. In other words, when we smile we cannot feel angry, for instance, at the exact moment we are smiling! It appears to be physiologically impossible."

The fact of the matter is that insecurity is really fear in disguise; fear that we're not good enough, not pretty enough, not smart enough, not successful or worthy or rich or attractive or tall or short enough.

I'll never forget how insecure I felt before getting braces at 15. Even though I was able to con my way into Run DMC's dressing room and flash Russell Simmons's business card to gain backstage access to one of the '80s best hip-hop concerts, those confident and blissful moments were few and far between. Inside I was second-guessing every move, every outfit, every hairstyle, every comment; all because of how the kids at school made me feel.

It's one thing to let others make you feel insecure; it's quite another when that insecurity spills over and takes over how you think about yourself. Why? Because we have enough negative thoughts every day; we don't need a single one more. Especially the kind that makes us so anxious we limit our lives.

That's right; insecurity is fear and fear kills hopes, dreams, thoughts, accomplishments and goals. When we are fearful, we doubt ourselves; when we doubt ourselves, we give up on things before we even try. Insecurity – fear – makes us avoid asking out that cute guy in Accounting, makes us skip speaking to the boss about that big promotion or even trying out for that new job in the first place. Don't let a simple thing like your smile rob you of life's greatest opportunities.

Next stop: CONFIDENCE!

A-List Advice:

By being prouder of your smile you become less insecure. In fact, regardless of how your smile looks right now, I have found that it is impossible to feel insecure when you are smiling.

More Smiles, More Confidence

It's a pretty simple equation, don't you think? Less insecurity = more confidence. But for some of us, our old insecurities are hard to get rid of, no matter how much we try. A lot of my patients who try to overcome their insecurity on their own don't realize how hard a struggle it can be until I point out that they've been fighting with one hand tied behind their back.

That's right; trying to lose your insecurity on your own is hard enough, but leaving your smile the way it is only makes things harder. Think how much easier life would be if you had a brighter, whiter smile while you were working on your self-confidence. Why, it would almost be like cheating! (It's okay; this is one time when I say it's okay to cheat.)

Previous consumer studies have proven that a beautiful smile will make you more attractive. But according to research conducted by Beall Research & Training of Chicago, a new smile will make you appear more intelligent, interesting, successful and wealthy to others as well.

None of these traits are possible without having confidence! Think about how your favorite celebrity, musician or movie star strides confidently out onto the red carpet before some movie premiere, concert or awards show. Watch them carefully next time and see how broadly, how widely they smile; notice how the wider, brighter and more naturally they smile, the more confident, radiant and cool they appear. This is no accident; great smiles breed superior confidence!

Dr. Anne Beall, a social psychologist and market research professional, carried out the independent study on behalf of the American Academy of Cosmetic Dentistry (AACD). Pictures of eight individuals were shown to 528 Americans, a statistically valid cross section of the population.

"To have large gains in how successful, intelligent, interesting and wealthy patients appeared after cosmetic dentistry caught even us by surprise," explains the American Academy of Cosmetic Dentistry (AACD). "We've been telling people that a beautiful smile was a great investment in their futures. Now we have independent evidence."

A-List Advice:

Less insecurity = more confidence.

What Confident People Know – and Enjoy

9 Gifts You'll Find in This Book – For Your Career, For Your Life, For Yourself

I would like to finish this section with a special kind of wish list; an "A-List" wish list, to be precise. But this isn't a list of things you give to others on their birthday or during the holidays – this is a wish list designed **specifically for you**. These are your gifts; the most important kind of all – the gifts you give yourself.

We all know how important teamwork can be; how vital a knowledgeable mentor or passionate co-worker can be to both our collective and individual success. The coach who gets you out of bed early every morning and out on that track – when it's the last thing in the world you want to do. The professor who grills you on every question as if it's the most important on the test – because it could just be.

But at the end of the day, it's you standing on that starting line – you've got to run the race for yourself; it's you with the # 2 pencil in your hand – you've got to pass or fail that test on your own merits. Others can help us on this path called "life," but it's up to us to take each individual step on our own – for better or worse.

If I were making "the list before the list," I would say that personal accountability is the prequel to the 10 items I'm about to offer you in this self-help book; you have to be ready to receive them, up for reading them and, most important of all, personally accountable for implementing them in your daily life; otherwise, they're all but useless.

Don't let the title of this book fool you: an A-List Smile is just as much a philosophy than a result. In other words, it's the gift of confidence – and as we all know, confidence doesn't just start at 9 and end at 5. It resides in the very core of your being; confidence is the wellspring from which all our good ideas and positive actions spring.

So an A-List Smile can reverberate throughout every area of your life: work, home, play, investing, health, wellness, even romance and sex! When you have an A-List Smile you have more than just straight, white teeth to go with your briefcase or pinstripe suit – you have the unbreakable trait of self-confidence – and with that you can truly conquer any world you desire.

So with that understanding in mind, below please find the ***9 Gifts You'll Find in This Book*** – *For Your Career, For Your Life, For Yourself*:

Gift # 1:

Information

As busy people in a busy world, we all know how important solid, timely and accurate information can be. If we are to move forward, quickly and with confidence, we first need accurate, credible and above all *timely* information on which to base our most vital business decisions.

Why are print newspaper readers and magazine subscribers dwindling drastically in favor of online news and periodical sources? Simple: because we can no longer wait a month, a week or in some cases even a day to get our information.

We want it **now, fast, quick and easy**.

5 Steps to a Hollywood A-List Smile is designed to be all of the above – **now, fast, quick and easy** – and then some. I know that when I read a book like this I want the fat cut, the gristle trimmed, the seasonings sprinkled in all the right places in just the right amount and the information served piping hot and ready to digest!

And that is what I offer you: camera-ready, use-today advice, information, celebrity anecdotes and expert tips to help you get, keep and maintain an A-List Smile so that you can truly enjoy all that business, life and the world around you has to offer.

Gift # 2:

Flexibility

Tom Peters, noted business expert and author of – among a dozen or more other titles – ***Thriving on Chaos**: Handbook for a Management Revolution*, once wrote, "Smile if it kills you. The physiology of smiling diffuses a lot of anger and angst. It makes your body and soul feel better."

As someone who has the art of the smile down to a science, I can tell you that Peters is 200% right; smiling *does* make "your body and soul feel better." Many of us think that smiling is a purely physical act, completely unrelated to our emotions. But as the expert quotes, research and opinions I've gathered throughout my career – and sprinkle within the pages of this book – prove, the physical can affect the emotional, and vice versa.

5 Steps to a Hollywood A-List Smile gives you the gift of flexibility; you do not have to be tied into the rugged grind of plowing through your days all doom and gloom, head down, sleeves rolled up and permanent frown affixed to your smiling face. Yes, I know; we all realize the harm in a "fixed smile," that painted-on grin that remains the same through good times and bad, hard meetings and easy ones; the smile that means little and hurts much.

That is NOT an A-List Smile; the smile I'm talking about is honest, sincere, flexible and authentic. You smile because you mean it, because it feels good, because you're genuinely happy about your appearance and confident in your skills to get the job – any job – done in a way that fosters success instead of failure. Flexibility means freedom to respond to any given situation in a positive manner; quickly, competently and with calm assurance that will complete the task.

When we lack confidence in ourselves – due in large part to our appearance and how preoccupied we've become with a few physical "faults" – we restrict ourselves from being open or accessible to new opportunities. Unfortunately, that is the direct opposite of flexibility in the workplace.

Gift # 3:

Speed

Think of how much more you could accomplish in a day if you were more confident in your own skills and accomplishments and less hesitant about whether or not you are qualified for this promotion or that seat at the negotiating table. Fear of certain situations or repercussions can be a necessary part of staying safe, but fear of your own talents and gifts does more harm than good – in and out of the office.

Kenneth Goode, author of *How to Win What You Want*, explains his secret for success through this simple strategy: "Get out of bed forcing a smile. You may not smile because you are cheerful; but if you will force yourself to smile you'll... be cheerful because you smile."

I often tell my patients that smiling is a habit; we get habits by practicing them until they are second nature. I know you may need some convincing to appreciate the true, positive power of the smile. The most I can offer you is the gift of practicing your own A-List Smile until it's second nature – then you can literally feel for yourself how much harder it is to be negative, fearful or overly cautious when you've got a smile on your face.

And what of speed, my third gift on this ultimate wish list? Speed is a natural occurrence of habit; when we feel confident we make decisions more easily – and much more rapidly. The more comfortable we get with making decisions rapidly, the more decisions we can make and with more confidence.

We often confuse speed with haste, but I am by no means suggesting you be hasty, rash or careless – only offering the choice that true confidence gives you in acting with positive, passionate, precise and prompt decisions when all around you fear and distrust is costing the competition dearly.

Gift # 4:

Understanding

One of the greatest gifts I can give you in this book is not to tell you that I understand where you've come from, where you're going or even what you're going through, but I *can* give you the gift of sharing **the spirit of understanding** that comes from helping thousands of people over the years get, keep and maintain an A-List Smile.

Although I'm known in New York and Los Angeles as "dentist to the stars," I have treated patients from all walks of life; from entry-level employees looking to get a leg up to busy and fearful executives looking to stay in the game. They all sit in my chair seeking a brighter, healthier smile as a way to accentuate and convey a stronger sense of pride and confidence – to their peers, their mentors, their supervisors, their employees, their family, their friends – to themselves.

This inner feeling of pride and accomplishment brings to mind my favorite quote from Emilie Barnes, author of ***Good Manners for Every Occasion***: *How to Look Smart and Act Right*: "Smile at someone and find something worth laughing about. As the laughter permeates your life, the spirit of celebration will take root in your heart."

Gift # 5:

Compassion

Compassion is not just a gift we give to others; it's a gift we give to ourselves, and I am proud to include it on this list of gifts I'm eager to share with you. We often see compassion as weakness, but in all the executives I've had pass through my chair over the years I remember those who struck me as the most compassionate were also those I respected the most and, not coincidentally, those who seemed to have found the most success in their own careers.

Our careers are defined by two things: our words and our deeds. Throughout each busy day, we are continually saying and doing things that move us forward or backward – depending on the effectiveness of those very words and deeds. Think how what you say and do affects others – this is a gift *5 Steps to a Hollywood A-List Smile* offers you a thousand times over.

For it's not just how big a deal you pull off at the negotiating table or how big an account you land on that next business trip that determines your future success – it's how you treat the people you work with, every day, who produce the products or ideas or creations that you're negotiating over or dealing with.

As Maya Angelou once wrote, "If you only have one smile in you, give it to the people you love. Don't be surly at home and then go out in the street and start grinning 'Good Morning' at total strangers." In other words, don't save your compassion for the bigwigs or your next big client; there's plenty to go around, so why not spread it around with the people you see every single day?

When you truly have, and continue to covet, the feelings of pride and self-worth inherent in an A-List Smile, you *will* find that you are truly a more passionate person because of how good you feel deep down inside.

Gift # 6:

Experience

"Of all the things you wear, your expression is the most important." So says Janet Lane, author of *Natural Light*. How true; but I do more than appreciate this quote – I live it every single day, in and out of the office.

In fact, I have been using, teaching, sharing and benefiting from an A-List Smile ever since my high school senior class voted me "Prettiest Smile." Over the years my own A-List Smile has allowed me to enter into arenas formerly forbidden to me and to overcome obstacles I might not have even attempted had I still been that shy little middle school girl so ashamed of her front teeth.

I know firsthand the benefits of an A-List Smile; it has brought me not only great success, but the kind of self-confidence that is truly unshakeable. My smile, and the confidence it has brought me, has allowed me to try new ventures and cross-promote my franchise in ways I never deemed possible.

Just think, as a girl from Flint, Michigan (where, as director Michael Moore frequently highlights in his films, the odds of surviving are stacked against you) I've been able start my first practice on the most expensive street in America – New York's 57th Street. After that came the building of my celebrity clientele, then becoming a spokesperson for the second largest pharmaceutical company in the world, GlaxoSmithKline (maker of Aquafresh), to starting a second dental practice in Los Angeles.

Being licensed to practice dentistry in the States of New York and California, I am able to work on both coasts providing cosmetic dentistry services backstage, at entertainment studios, on photo shoots and in corner offices "from sea to shining sea." All because I took the steps to get an A-List Smile!

Gift # 7:

Success

English poet, essayist and man of letters Joseph Addison once wrote, "What sunshine is to flowers, smiles are to humanity. They are trifles, to be sure; but, scattered along life's pathway, the good they do is inconceivable."

What does doing good have to do with doing well? In this day and age, few of us can dispute the fact that more and more businesses are becoming more and more socially responsible. From clothes manufacturers treating their employers more humanely to big-box retailers reaching fair trade agreements with foreign countries to ALL companies responding to their impact on the global environment, more than ever doing good IS the secret to doing well.

5 Steps to a Hollywood A-List Smile is about CHANGE, first and foremost; change for you, change for your appearance, change for your attitude, change for your company – change for the better. Don't be fooled by thinking that your appearance doesn't matter; it is no longer vanity to think of how you look as important to how you face the world, but a necessity to help express how you feel – and who you are – sooner, faster and more effectively than ever before.

When you feel good about yourself, you do better in every aspect of your life. When your performance improves, you become more successful – when you become more successful, your value is enhanced. Best of all, when this success and value comes from deep within you, it is that much easier to contribute to the greater good by being happy, confident and strong where it matters the most – deep inside.

Gift # 8:

Motivation

Mother Teresa once said, "Let us always meet each other with a smile, for the smile is the beginning of love." I think it's important as we move forward through this book to remember that success is empty – at any level, be it entry-level or the corner office – without love in your heart.

5 Steps to a Hollywood A-List Smile reminds us of why we got into whatever business it is we got into however long ago in the first place. Was it to change the world? Create a new product? Travel the globe? Introduce a new concept to help revitalize an old idea? Whatever your reasons, we all know that where we end up can often be a long, long way from where we started – even from the destination we first had in mind.

Sometimes obstacles become opportunities and road blocks become watershed moments; other times such interruptions to your career or life's plan can downright derail, deflate and depress you. What I offer in this book is the joy of discovering – perhaps even reconnecting with – the unblemished sense of raw motivation you had inside when you first embarked on your own particular path.

Together we can rediscover the enthusiasm that brought you to the starting line and, by retracing your steps, we can also reenergize that sense of motivation that might have been lacking in your current business and personal dealings.

Remember that an A-List Smile is more than just our teeth, lips, gums and facial muscles; it's a concept for building self-confidence in every aspect of your life. I find that, in my busy dental practice, motivation is a gift we can all use a lot more of – and a lot more often!

Gift # 9:

Memory

Everyone loves to smile, giggle, beam, guffaw, grin and smirk. What's so sad about this little maxim is that **most of us don't remember to**

do any of the above as much as we used to. Discovery Health reports that, in fact, "By the time a child reaches nursery school, he or she will laugh about 300 times a day. Adults laugh an average of 17 times a day."

Where do you fall in that national average? Over 17 times a day? Under? Way, way, WAY under? What is it about adulthood that saps the smile from us? How do, over the years, we go from laughing, smiling, giggling and grinning 300 times a day to beaming only a fraction of that number in our adult lives?

We could go on for pages about the reasons why we smile less often as adults than we did as children – but my final gift to you is not a question, but an answer: I will help you reach back into the joys of your childhood years and remember what it's like to laugh for the sake of laughing – to smile just because it's another great day outside your window, full of opportunities, joy, possibility and success.

A-List Advice:

This isn't a list of things you give to others on their birthday or during the holidays – this is a wish list designed ***specifically for you****. These are your gifts; the most important kind of all – the gifts you give yourself.*

"A smile is one of the first features that you see. It's important for artists to have a beautiful smile when performing in front of the camera."

~ Ciarra

Step 3:

Prepare for Your A-List Smile

"Wear a smile and have friends; wear a scowl and have wrinkles."

~ George Eliot

Speaking of gifts, an A-List Smile is the gift you give yourself. Isn't it time you treated yourself to something that could change your entire life, give you more success, more confidence, more companionship and even add longer, healthier years to your life?

I'm so happy we're finally at ***Step 3**: How to Get Started With Your A-List Smile*. Why? Because I finally get to use the phrase all dentists everywhere love to use: **Time to put your money where your mouth is!** That's right; here is where we finally get started in the process of securing for you an A-List Smile you can be proud of for years, maybe even decades, to come.

I get excited when patients come in to consult with me about their smiles, no matter what shape they're currently in; that's because I know what's in store for them: namely more confidence, security, poise, professionalism, health, symmetry and just plain happiness. So as we go through this third step of the process, I hope that you, too, feel energized about the direction you're headed.

After all, this is a time for change, hope, optimism and satisfaction. You are about to embark upon a journey that will change the way you feel about not just your smile, but your very self. No matter how long you've been unsatisfied with your smile or unhappy with yourself, now you've decided to take action – and this is where you start.

Take time out during this vital third step to consider not just how much you want to do about your smile but even when you want to do it and why. For instance, you may want to wait until summer if you're a teacher because you'll have more time off to recuperate and get used to your new smile, or you may want to wait until winter because you spend more time indoors.

Smiling isn't just a physical act, it's a habit we either get into or grow out of. So this section is all about building strong habits, be they in your mouth or a little farther upstairs in your brain. Remember, for a smile to last a lifetime, you've got to build a lifetime of good habits.

Here is where we begin:

A-List Advice:

Get into the habit of noticing good smiles, be they on the street, in a magazine or movie poster or on TV. Don't just notice them, either, but pay attention to what makes them an A-List Smile; by noticing what makes other smiles so attractive, you'll be all the more ready to design your own.

First Things First:

SMILE!

The first thing I want you to do as we continue our journey together toward your brand new smile is to get in practice; that's right: SMILE. When psychiatrists begin treating their phobia patients, they often encourage them to take "baby steps" toward overcoming whatever it is they're afraid of.

In other words, if their patient is afraid of heights, a psychiatrist will tell them to start by climbing a stepladder, then a regular ladder, then a flight of stairs, then two, then three. You get my point. Well, maybe you have a phobia of smiling brought on by years of insecurity, negativity and self-doubt; all through this chapter I want you to remember to smile. Just… SMILE.

It might be hard at first, and it could feel funny sitting there reading this and just suddenly breaking out in a smile, but if you really want to know the first place to begin your journey to an A-List Smile, it's not in a dentist's chair or at the library researching various dental professionals, it's between your very own lips.

Test Your Smile Reflexes

To help make smiling more of a habit and less of an annual event, take my Test Your Smile Reflexes Quiz. It's simple; no grades, just gut-check reactions. First, answer the following few groups of questions:

When you meet someone new, do you…

- Shake their hand carefully and look them up and down?
- Try to impress them with your importance?
- Smile openly at them and give a warm handshake?

When you greet an old friend, do you…

- Say, "Wow, I wouldn't have recognized you! What did you do to your hair?"
- Feel guilty you haven't been in touch for awhile.
- Smile broadly and hug them.

When you walk into your office building in the morning, do you…

- Hurry through the lobby and jump on the elevator?
- Feel so worried about work you don't look around?
- Feel energized and smile at the people you pass?

When you leave your office at the end of the day and say "goodnight" to coworkers, do you….

- Run toward the elevator, throwing your farewells over your shoulder?
- Only say "goodnight" to your special buddies?
- Smile graciously at your colleagues and wish them a good evening?

When you make a public presentation, do you…

- Look as serious as possible so everyone will take you seriously?
- Speak rapidly and feel self-conscious about how you look and sound?
- Look your colleagues in the eye and share your enthusiasm for your subject by smiling and drawing them in?

Of course, these are only a few examples of how so many of us behave unthinkingly during the day. Time and again, we throw away opportunities to smile and to share our good mood with others. Here are some other great opportunities to smile; so read the following list of daily, weekly or regular events. Next to each item, write "S" for every time you're likely to smile and "F" for every time you're likely to frown:

_____ **Pick up the kids from school**
_____ **Dine with friends and family**
_____ **Answer your phone**
_____ **Reapply your makeup**
_____ **Brush your teeth**
_____ **Get up in the morning**
_____ **Go to bed at night**
_____ **Get into or off of the elevator with people**
_____ **Get into or out of your car**
_____ **Open a door for someone**
_____ **Hear your favorite song**

If you had more "F" answers than "S" answers, give yourself a simple goal; write down the events that made you mark "F" next to them on a scratch sheet of paper; fold it and put it in your purse and/or wallet. Take it out from time to time, every day at lunch, say, or just before leaving work, to remind yourself of those things that normally cause you to do anything but smile. Every week, focus on one item on your list – such as "During a presentation" or "Open a door for someone" – and consciously work on smiling whenever you run into that situation.

When smiling at the beginning of a presentation or while opening the door becomes second nature, cross that item off and move onto the next item on your list. As you can see, there are as many occasions for you to smile as there are reasons for you to smile in the first place. So don't wait to find a dentist to start the process of getting a head start on your A-List Smile.

If you're smiling while you're reading this, you've already begun!

A-List Advice:

Get in the habit of smiling every time you walk past a mirror. At home, in some random lobby, in the car or at work, this will help you get ready for your A-List Smile. And don't worry, it's not vanity – it's therapy!

The Top 10 Dental Mistakes People Make That Can Ruin Their Smiles

As a dentist, I'm not the most popular person in the world. But I've worked hard to change the perception of dentists as "worldwide pain-inflicters" to something a lot more positive: "universal confidence-boosters"!

Going to the dentist may not be fun, but I try really hard to make it so. Having a bright, straight, confident smile can change your world in many ways, and I've made it my mission to share that information with people by trying to make going to the dentist something to look forward to rather than avoid.

I've always said that some people don't think about their dentist enough; other people think about their dentist too much! Here are the **Top 10 Dental Mistakes People Make That Can Ruin Their Smiles** (in reverse order):

10.) Sticking with a dentist/dental office that you don't enjoy visiting twice a year.

9.) Trying to whiten your own teeth with "real" bleach! (Believe it or not, I've had patients who've tried this!)

8.) Not getting enough – or any – fluoride in your system to fight cavities.

7.) Not paying attention to the hidden sugar in your food and drinks.

6.) Using a hard or medium bristled toothbrush in hopes of getting better cleaning results.

5.) Trying to "mask" bad breath with gum, mints or tongue strips.

4.) Not brushing your teeth before you go to bed.

3.) Daring to think that you can skip flossing every day!

2.) Avoiding dental treatment because your insurance told you that you couldn't get it done because of THEIR rules.

1.) Saying to yourself, "My teeth are fine. I don't need to see a dentist."

Being a Consumer First, A Patient Second

One of the things that happens when patients sit in my chair is that they tend to feel overwhelmed, intimidated – or both. But this limits the dentist-patient relationship because then we're not working on equal footing. Sometimes, for instance, patients tell me **what they think I want to hear** when, actually, the truth is a much better instrument to help me form a diagnoses for **what they really need**.

I suppose it's natural to feel this way. For so long, growing up, we were taught to "listen to the doctor" and "don't interfere." Now, of course, modern physician-patient relationships are built on mutual trust and the free exchange of information. It's the doctor who wants to listen to you and, if you don't "interfere," how will you ever get the quality care you really deserve?

The best way to cast off those old-fashioned stereotypes concerning the physician-patient relationship is to think of yourself not as a patient, but as a customer. After all, you're paying for a product or procedure, so it only makes sense that you should act the same way in the dentist's office as you do when you walk into a store.

You wouldn't walk into Best Buy and choose the first big-screen TV you see on the sales floor, would you? Of course not, so why would you take what your dental provider says at face value, either?

Just as there are many different styles and makes of big-screen televisions – flat panel versus widescreen, digital versus beta, etc. – the path to an A-List Smile is filled with many different options, varieties, comfort levels and criteria. When you think of your dentist as a **retailer** and yourself as a **customer**, you will feel much better about making just the right selection for yourself.

Here are some quick ways to do just that:

- **Ask questions**: Don't be uncomfortable asking for more information if you didn't quite comprehend what your dentist was saying the first time around. If you don't understand something – a dental term, a price quote, a recovery time or even the name of the procedure itself – ask, and ask again, until you do. A good dental provider will always encourage questions from a patient-customer, not discourage them.
- **Verify approval**: You should know what – and where – your dentist is approved to practice. Most states have a dental board and website where you can check the status of a dentist's license, whether it's current or suspended. Some sites offer information about malpractice suits as well.
- **Note education and affiliations**: Legitimate questions for you to ask your dentist include what dental school they attended, if they're certified and if they're taking continuing education classes. Associations for dentists and cosmetic professionals include the American Academy of Cosmetic Dentistry, the Academy of General Dentistry and the American Dental Association.
- **Know the makers of the hardware**: Because veneers, partials and implants are ordered by dentists, not made by them, be sure to ask about the laboratories and ceramists your dentist might be using. You can then do some research back home to make sure the lab(s) your dentist uses is up to industry standards.
- **Be knowledgeable**: The best way to know what questions to ask is not to think about them on the way home from the dentist's office, but to be informed *before* you go to your appointment. To avoid that "aha" moment on the way home when you think about what you should have asked if only you'd been better prepared, write down your questions beforehand

and bring them with you. This means doing your homework (see the following section for pointers on this) and coming to the dentist's office prepared.

- **Shop around**: Just because you're thinking of going with one dental provider over another – or a whole list of others – doesn't mean you can't still shop around for the information you need. Explore other dentists' websites, blogs, newsletters and articles until you find what you are looking for. Maybe your dental provider is great hands-on but not so great with updating his or her website with the latest information on dentistry; go to another dental website to find more information on the procedures you're considering. Is it acceptable to do this? You bet it is! Better yet, it's advisable!

A-List Advice:

Don't be afraid to ask someone "Who is your dentist?" when you spot a person on the street with an A-List Smile. In my experience, people love to show their smiles off and, what's more, brag on the dentist who helped them.

Be a "Smile Sponge":

Get Informed, Stay Informed

As you begin your journey_for a qualified dental provider to assist you with getting an A-List Smile, you may feel a little overwhelmed at the prospect. The choices can leave you breathless and the sheer volume of information you discover can seem extremely daunting.

So many dental providers, so little time!

But not only is time on your side, information is power – and the more you know about local dental providers and the products and procedures they offer, the less intimidated you'll feel – and the more powerful you'll become.

The surest way to gain knowledge is through information, and that means to **get and stay** informed; but there's more to it than that. There is no substitute for knowledge, and in addition to what you read in this book it's important to do research on your own. In fact, there are two main ways to go about this very process:

- **Get Informed**: Learn everything you can about what you need to do to start working on an A-List Smile. Reading this book is a great start, but so is locating a dentist, looking up various procedures and actually educating yourself to understand them, as well as getting to know the various products and procedures on the market and how they work. Be a "smile sponge" and soak up as much information as you can.

- **Stay Informed**: Staying informed means going above and beyond what you already know. You have a list of doctors who might be a good fit for you? Great. Now learn more about them, such as where their office is located, how many people they have on staff and are they board certified. In other words, take what you know a little farther and keep up with any new developments, like a special offer by one of the dentists on your list, a change of address or even a new procedure you've read about and want to ask him or her to explain to you.

A-List Advice:

Don't skimp on the research; I've devoted an entire step to getting started with your smile because research is so important I decided it needed its own chapter. Remember, these are important decisions you're making and research merely makes you better informed.

How to Find the Right Dental Provider for Your A-List Smile

No step of the process for getting an A-List Smile is more important than finding the right dental provider for you. Note that I didn't say the most expensive, the nicest, or even the closest dental provider (these should not be the determining factors), only the right one – for you.

This may mean someone who "gets" you, who understands you, who makes you feel warm and fuzzy whenever you walk into his or her office. It may mean the dental provider with the most degrees, the fanciest office or the biggest staff. It may even mean someone in the next town over – or right next to your office building.

Like deciding what makes an A-List Smile or which products you'll need to obtain it, choosing your dental provider is entirely personal; it's also a difficult choice. You can't simply open up the yellow pages, flip to "dentists" and pick the first listing you see. You'll need to do a little – and in some cases a whole lot – of research first.

Fortunately, this handy list will give you plenty of places to start:

- **Family, Friends and Focus Groups**: Does your sister have a great smile? How about your mother-in-law, your neighbor, your cousin or your best friend? Where did they get it? Don't know? Why not ask? You want to find a dentist you can trust, so you should start by asking the people you trust. These can be family members, friends or your own personal "focus group" of colleagues at work or where you go to school.

- **Is There a Doctor in the House?** We often overlook them these days – perhaps because we don't see them as often as we used to – but your family doctor can be a wealth of medical information, even when it comes to choosing a dentist. Ask your doctor and/or nurses who they might recommend; you might be surprised by how consistent their advice is on the matter.
- **Church and Social Groups**: If you are a social person and attend church regularly, you are in luck; these wonderful places to meet and congregate are also valuable pools of information when it comes to various local and community resources, including dental professionals.
- **Online Works**: The internet can be a great place to look up the names of dental providers as your gather them from the above sources. Many modern dental professionals have websites that not only explain the various products and procedures they offer, but even let you know a little bit more about them, personally speaking. You can also find articles or opinions written by your prospective dental provider online, and many user boards offer critiques and testimonials of the provider in question.
- **Offline Does Too**: But don't forget to continue your search offline as well. If you have managed to do a considerable amount of research online, combine it with some offline "field trips," if you will. For instance, maybe you're really in favor of a certain dental provider because their office is very impressive. Great; super. Print their address and drive there. Is it the same building, grounds and manicured lawns as they portrayed on their website? Sometimes people use stock footage for their websites and you might find yourself in a less than professional office building or strip mall. So be careful of doing all of your research online; what you see isn't always what you get.
- **The Better Business Bureau**: As you start gathering names of dental professionals who might be best suited to give you your A-List Smile, be sure to "clear" them with the Better Business Bureau. Make sure that your dental provider of choice has a

clean bill of health on the BBB website, www.bbb.org, to make sure that everyone on your list deserves to be there.

A-List Advice:

Keep a running list of the best dental providers in your area, based on your exhaustive research. Go down the list and compare/contrast the dental providers; make a chart and list all the procedures and products they offer. When your search is over, your dental provider should be at the top of this list.

Time is on Your Side; Don't Rush into Anything

As we move forward through these sections it is important to remember that knowledge, understanding and research are key to making quality decisions about your dental care and getting an A-List Smile. Knowing what's on the market today will give you options that you may not even realize exist.

I often take high-tech and cutting-edge procedures for granted, but was reminded the other day of how little people really know about all these products and procedures on the market today. "Dr. Austin," said one gentleman in his mid-40s, "what you've just told me is amazing; why, I haven't thought about doing anything to my teeth since I got my braces off nearly thirty years ago!"

So remember that even if you think your smile is beyond hope, or your specific problem beyond fixing, or even a simple procedure is beyond your budget, think again! Slow down, take your time and read these sections carefully because the answer to your problem could be just around the corner. (Or, in this case, the next page!)

Of course, it wasn't always this way. Once upon a time, dentists and other members of the medical field were revered and well-rewarded for their skills. Patients, and money, were both plentiful and student loans were quickly paid off, as were mortgages and fancy cars. Today, however, there are more and more dental providers on every block and more and more liability and malpractice insurance premiums to pay for every dentist.

Unfortunately, instead of concentrating on honing their craft and personalizing their service to meet the demands of their patients, some dental providers have become more like salesmen, providing not only regular cleanings but also pushing – and pushing hard – procedures and products a patient may not need or, if they might eventually need them, may not be quite ready for just yet.

I had a patient come in not long ago whose teeth were in pretty poor shape. Although I knew it had been awhile since he'd been to the dentist, when I asked him how long it had been he responded with a "why" instead of a "when" answer.

He explained, "I've been to three dentists in the last six years and every single one of them was a high-pressure sales experience. One wanted me to get braces; another practically demanded I use his – and only his – whitening program and get veneers. The last one wanted to charge me separately to clean my upper and lower teeth; at $150 a pop!"

I understood his frustration. Know that what I am sharing with you in this section is NOT a high-pressure sales job or a way to make more money for myself, my competitors or my colleagues. That is what is so important about a book like this one; the more you know, the sooner you recognize when something is necessary or a luxury. The more informed you are, the better decisions you'll make.

And one of the first things you need to know when preparing to get your A-List Smile is that (in most instances), **time is on your side**. Yes, your routine cleanings need to be performed twice annually and cavities need to be filled but, barring various medical procedures that need to be done to protect your health, the assorted cosmetic products and procedures I'll outline in Step 4 can be done on your own time, at your own leisure.

Here are a few of the critical factors that may affect you when you have these procedures done:

- **Cost**: Price is often a factor when considering cosmetic dental procedures, particularly if you have an insufficient dental plan or even NO dental plan. While insurance carriers differ, even your estimated patient co-pay for those products and procedures that *are* covered can be expensive. So be aware of the costs involved and how they relate to your current savings and/or credit accounts. Speak with your dental provider openly and honestly about your cost concerns and explore all the options available to you concerning financing, paying over time, loans, etc.

- **Employment**: Work schedules are extremely important, particularly when you consider that the reason a lot of people want a more attractive A-List Smile has to do with seeking more confidence on and off the job site. If you are someone who travels frequently for their job, is a workaholic or doesn't have a lot of sick days or down time associated with your current job, then employment may be a big factor in when you can have your procedure. That is why it's important to know what, exactly, is involved with each product and procedure – see Step 4 – so you can know exactly how long you need to take off of work to recuperate, if any time is needed at all. If necessary, you may want to schedule your appointment on a Friday so that you can take the weekend to recover. For other procedures, you may need longer, or shorter, recovery times. Either way, the more you know, the better you can prepare for scheduling in advance.
- **Health**: Your health is of the utmost importance when scheduling any dental procedure, be it surgical or non-surgical. Anytime anesthesia, needles or appliances are involved, you need to be free of sickness. That is why your dental provider wants to know so much about your physical health the first time you make a visit to his or her office. Sometimes, medical clearance is needed by your medical doctor before we begin dental procedures. Even things like whether or not you smoke, exercise, drink alcohol or take drugs can affect how your dental provider treats you. So if your health needs to improve before you have any products or procedures done, don't rush it; your body, and your dentist, will thank you for waiting!

A-List Advice:

Invest in a calendar – no matter how late in the year it is – and look ahead in the months remaining to determine the best time for your procedure. My patients find that seeing the dates in question in black and white on a calendar really helps them make better decisions as to when, exactly, to have their procedures done.

Surgical Versus Non-surgical, a Personal Choice

Every one of my patients has what I call a "unique risk threshold." In other words, some have a high tolerance for dental procedures, others are particularly squeamish – and still others fall somewhere in between.

One thing I've learned is that you can never tell by looking; I've had huge musclemen faint at the first sign of a needle and on the opposite side of the spectrum I've had teeny-tiny women easily take on much more surgical and involved procedures.

The fact of the matter is, having a surgical versus a non-surgical procedure is your choice; nobody else's. Don't let anyone, let alone your dental provider, talk, bully or pressure you into doing something you don't need to do or, even worse, something you absolutely, positively don't *want* to do.

That said, let's talk openly and honestly about the various pros and cons of invasive versus non-invasive procedures:

Surgical Procedures

In my office, as in many dental offices around the country, I offer a variety of procedures with varying degrees of intensity, including more involved procedures like tooth extractions, implants, and gum surgery.

Let's talk about why surgical procedures may or may not be right for you:

- **Pros**: If your smile is really in need of an overhaul, for either cosmetic or even comfort reasons, surgery can perform a myriad of beneficial tasks to properly give you the effect you are looking for. It can actually provide drastic, life-changing results. Modern technology has also made surgery less painful, more effective and involving less recovery time than ever before.
- **Cons**: Surgery can be intimidating to a lot of people; sadly, this is something they may not be able to overcome when trying to obtain their A-List Smile. Recovery times can occasionally be painful and prolonged, though most involve only soreness for no more than 1-2 days.

The great news is that many dentists offer various sedation techniques that can make your dental procedure a breeze! You can choose to be mildly sedated but remain awake during the procedure with just laughing gas (nitrous oxide), your dentist can prescribe valium to keep you awake but more relaxed, or you can request IV sedation where you sleep during the procedure. Consult with your dentist and medical physician to see if you are a healthy candidate for sedation.

Non-surgical Procedures

There are a variety of non-surgical cosmetic dental procedures that can help you attain your A-List Smile. (See Step 4 for details.) For instance, procedures like Invisalign® Clear Braces, porcelain veneers, ZOOM!® Teeth Whitening and the Snap-On Smile® are all non-surgical procedures that require minimal invasion. Here we examine some of the pros and cons of non-surgical procedures:

- **Pros**: With non-surgical procedures, obviously, you don't have the anxiety, pain, or longer recovery times of surgery. Most non-surgical procedures are done on an outpatient basis, meaning you typically go home right after the procedure with minimal recovery. There is rarely, if any, pain involved; results are typically immediate and long-lasting.

- **Cons**: Some non-surgical procedures have limits. These procedures sometimes need maintenance and touching up more frequently than surgical procedures. Many times they only mask problems as opposed to correct or undo some of the more serious problems that surgery can handle.

The decision to have surgery or not have surgery is an entirely personal one. A good cosmetic dentist should present you with multiple options of treatment. Whatever you decide, know that there has never been a better time for dentistry. Today's products and technology are cutting edge, more effective and safer than ever before. If timing really IS everything, then you are getting an A-List Smile at just the right time!

A-List Advice:

Don't let others influence your final decision as you prepare for any procedure. By all means, listen to advice as it is given, but the final decision must be yours.

"Your smile helps you present your best you. You exude happiness when you smile."

~ Maxwell

Step 4:

Know What Products & Procedures Are On the Market, Which to Choose and How to Pay

"Before you put on a frown, make absolutely sure there are no smiles available."

~ Jim Beggs

Not every dental product and procedure on the market today is right for every patient who sits in my chair, and vice versa. In this section we will provide a consumer guide to teach you what products are out there today and how they can help you achieve that A-List Smile.

Here I weigh the pros and cons of each product and briefly list not only the price range of each procedure but also the duration and convenience of each. Price is not the only concern for my patients; many of them are busy working professionals and want to know exactly how long a procedure will take and when it will be ready for "their big debut" as well.

Below are the products and procedures that I recommend for readers to have an A-List Smile:

- **Smile Design**
    - o *Digital Radiography*
    - o *Digital "before and after" photos*
    - o *Stone replicas of your mouth*
    - o *Smile makeover results in wax*
- **Porcelain Veneers**
- **Invisalign® Clear Braces**
- **ZOOM!® Teeth Whitening**
- **Snap-On Smile®**
- **Porcelain Fillings**
- **Dental Implants**
- **Bonding**

For your convenience, I've broken all the products and procedures down in a very easy-to-follow style that quickly allows you to compare and contrast, so rest easy; (smile) shopping has never been so simple!

A-List Advice:

Even if you think you don't need veneers or tooth-colored fillings, be sure to read this entire chapter. Every procedure has some benefit, and it behooves you to be well-informed before you go to visit your dental expert of choice. After all, even if he or she recommends a procedure you don't want, at least this way you'll be qualified to tell them why!

What Is Smile Designing?

Cosmetic dentists are trained to design smiles; that is our art, our skill, our job and, for many of us, our passion. It is a process that begins by assessing the current condition of your teeth and learning what your cosmetic goals are during what is known as a "smile design consultation." Here is where the A-List Smile has its birth. Then, using smile design techniques, your dentist can craft new teeth, transforming your smile to A-List status.

Think your favorite celebrity was born looking drop-dead gorgeous? Think again; many famous A-Listers rely on celebrity dentists to help them look their best, both on and off the red carpet. From hip-hop stars like Kanye West and 50 Cent to movie stars like Tom Cruise and Cher to pop stars like Gwen Stefani and Christina Aguilera to athletes like Venus Williams to comedians like Chris Rock and even celebrity psychologist Dr. Joyce Brothers, famous people from every walk of life work hard to get their A-List smiles.

But you don't have to be famous to look the part; all you have to be is prepared! Part of creating an A-List Smile is being well-versed in smile design. For instance, in both my NY and LA offices, I have a full range of materials, equipment and techniques at my disposal—all the technology I need to create gorgeous, picture-perfect smiles.

Smile design technology includes intra-oral cameras and digital cameras for photographing your teeth, and digital software programs to give you a sneak preview of your future smile. You can either select your desired smile from photos or design books that your dentist has in the office or you can bring in photos.

Some patients bring photos of their own smiles when they were younger or happier with their smile. Others tend to bring in photos of a smile that they admire, like a famous smile (the "Julia Roberts Smile" is always a popular choice).

Your dentist can also make a stone replica of your teeth and design your desired smile in wax so you can see your new smile up close and personal in your hand. That's right, you no longer have to wait and wonder what your smile could look like if you choose cosmetic dentistry. Your cosmetic dentist can show you simulated images or wax replicas of your new smile before you invest the time and money in it.

A-List Advice:

Make sure that your dentist is trained in smile design. If he or she asks, "What's that?" when you ask, chances are they probably aren't!

Smile Makeover Treatments

Depending on your needs and goals, your dental expert may combine a number of different techniques to complete your A-List Smile makeover. Often, a simple smile makeover entails a professional teeth cleaning and teeth whitening with ZOOM! teeth-whitening. To correct minor problems with the position of your teeth, Invisalign clear braces or porcelain veneers may be recommended.

For more serious smile problems, you may need traditional braces, gum therapy, root canal surgery, extractions, implant placements, or crowns to complete your makeover. Your dental expert may suggest the Snap-On Smile, a removable dental appliance that gives you many of the benefits of a smile design with less cost and a smaller commitment of time. The beauty of the Snap-On Smile is that you can choose to wear it long term or for a short time as a "trial smile" before deciding if you want permanent makeover treatments.

The important thing to remember is to consult with your dental expert honestly, openly and exhaustively about just exactly what your options are. Regardless of your needs, your dental expert should be more than familiar with all of the above products and procedures – and so much more. If he or she isn't, ask them to recommend someone who is.

A-List Advice:

If you won't be using your regular dentist to help create your A-List Smile, be sure to research your new dentist thoroughly. I would start by asking for referrals or doing a Google search of the most renowned cosmetic dentist(s) in your area, then set up a consultation with your new dentist of choice to tour his or her office; if you don't like what you see and feel right away, continue searching until you find the dentist that you feel most comfortable with.

Porcelain Veneers

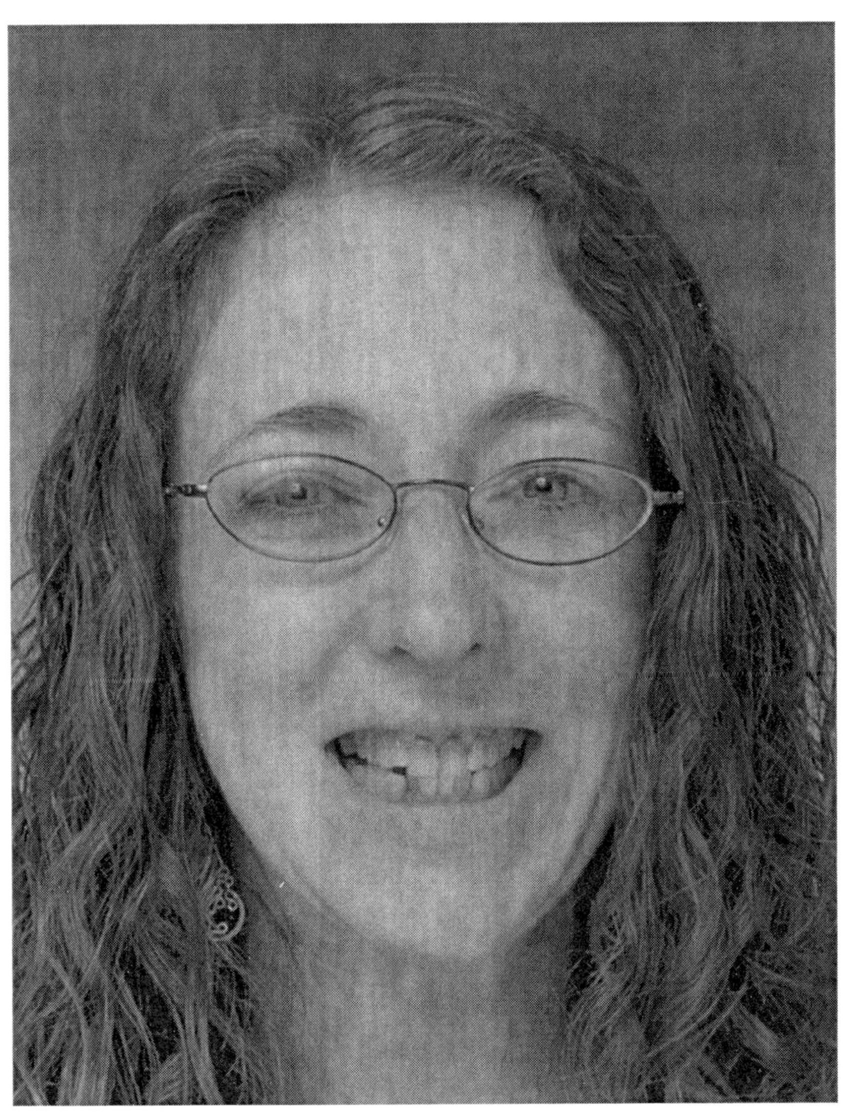

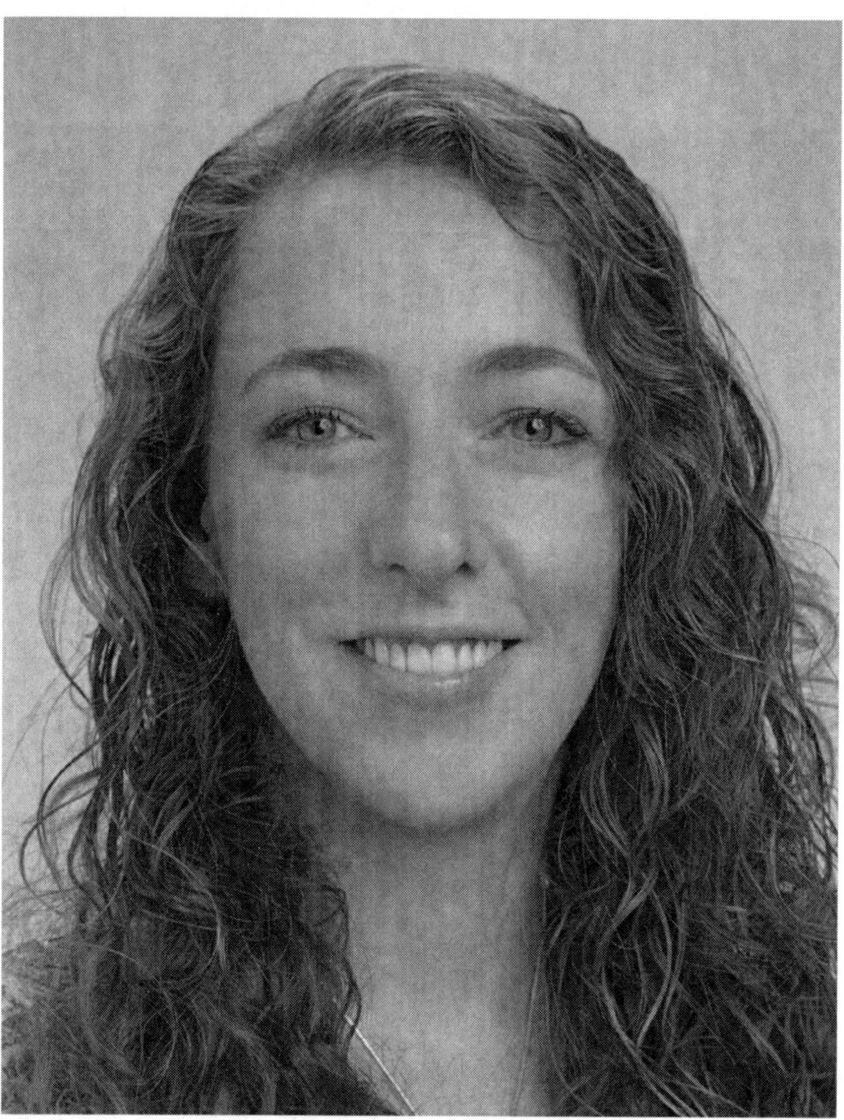

Elliot Yamin, former American Idol contestant and now bonafide pop star, took a lot of flack for his teeth before, during and after the hit TV show – and responded with great veneers that took his smile from the D-list straight to the red carpet! And Disney sensation and pop star Miley Cyrus helped bridge the gaps in her teeth by reportedly having veneers put on.

Other stars that have gotten veneers and have been in the media for it include Hillary Duff, rapper 50 Cent, singer Keyshia Cole, Lil Kim, Christina Aguilera and Chris Rock. Although not the most cost effective for those on a budget, veneers are THE procedure that can give you that Hollywood A-List Smile with guaranteed red carpet results.

What do they do? Porcelain veneers are excellent for restoring the appearance of teeth that have been damaged due to injury or that are discolored, chipped or misaligned. The color, shape, length and size of your teeth can be completely altered with high-quality porcelain veneers. Any dentist who is an expert in cosmetic dentistry can make you look younger and more attractive with porcelain veneers.

Porcelain veneers replace the enamel of your teeth by bonding to the front of each tooth. I compare them to "fake fingernails," but for the teeth. Like natural enamel, these thin, glass-like veneers are translucent and light-absorbing, which creates a natural and luminescent appearance. With porcelain veneers, you can have the beautiful, natural-looking smile you've always wanted.

How does the procedure work?

During your first office visit, your dentist will walk you through the various stages of your porcelain veneers procedure, allowing you to take an active role in designing your new smile. Your dentist may need to administer anesthesia depending on how much tooth structure has to be removed to achieve the desired results. Next, your teeth will be buffed and reshaped as needed. Generally only about half a millimeter of enamel will be removed.

A putty mold of your teeth will then be made in preparation for the laboratory ceramist to design and make your new porcelain teeth for bonding during your second office visit. The ceramist has to carefully hand sculpt each and every tooth to your desired color and shape that was selected during the smile design phase. Your dentist will complete your first visit by making temporary veneers to replace the enamel that was removed. These temporary veneers are made of acrylic and, if planned properly, can be made from the wax-up model of your new smile that was made during the smile design process to give you a sneak preview of your new smile.

During your second visit, your dentist will administer anesthesia to prepare you for the removal of your temporary veneers. Next, your new porcelain veneers will be fitted to your teeth with temporary glue for viewing your new smile.

You should look at your new smile from different angles, different sized mirrors, and under different lighting. In my office, I have my patients look first in a hand held mirror in the chair, then in a vanity mirror on the wall of the bathroom, and finally a full length mirror. The goal is to see the veneers under different scenarios to make sure that you like them, before they are permanently bonded to your teeth.

If there is something that you don't like about the veneers, you can request that the veneers be sent back to be remade to your specification at no additional cost. However, once they are bonded with permanent glue, the veneers are yours to keep and any changes that are requested may cost you handsomely. Upon your approval, your new porcelain veneers will be bonded permanently and polished to give you a beautiful, natural-looking smile.

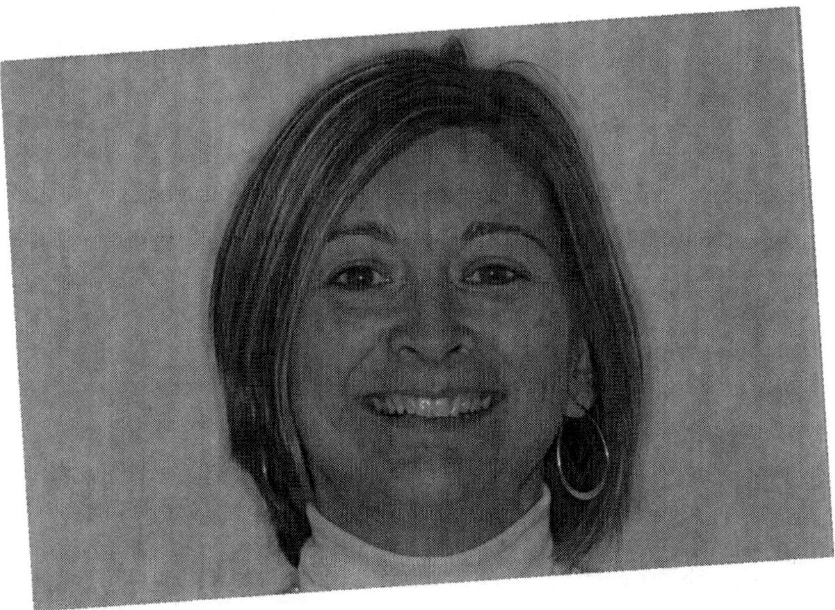

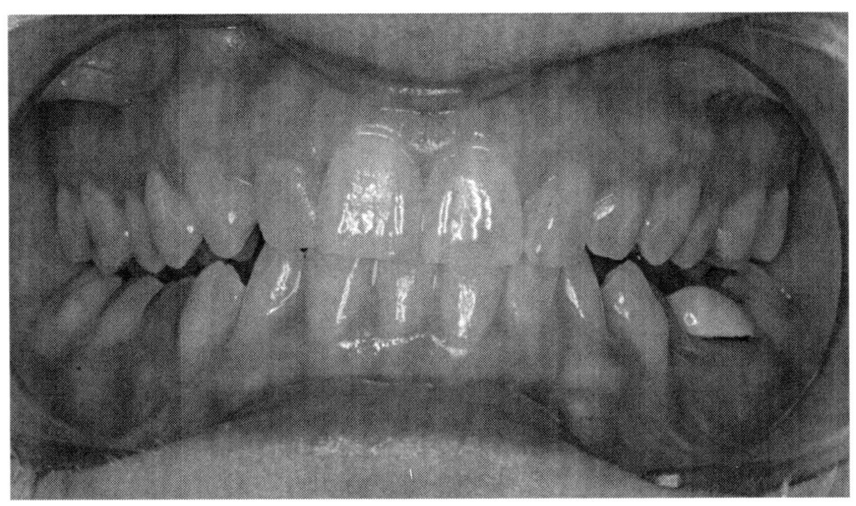

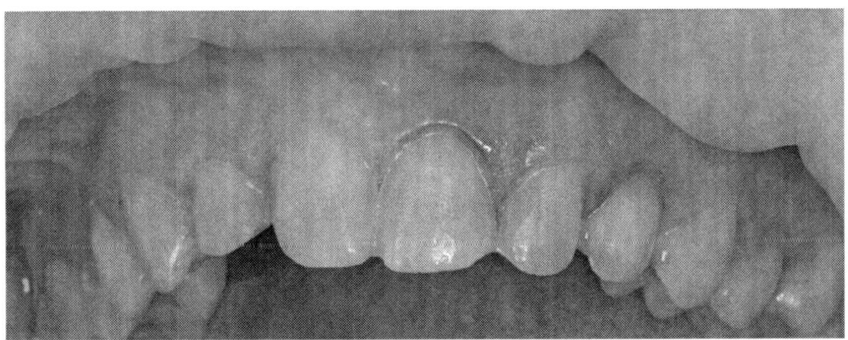

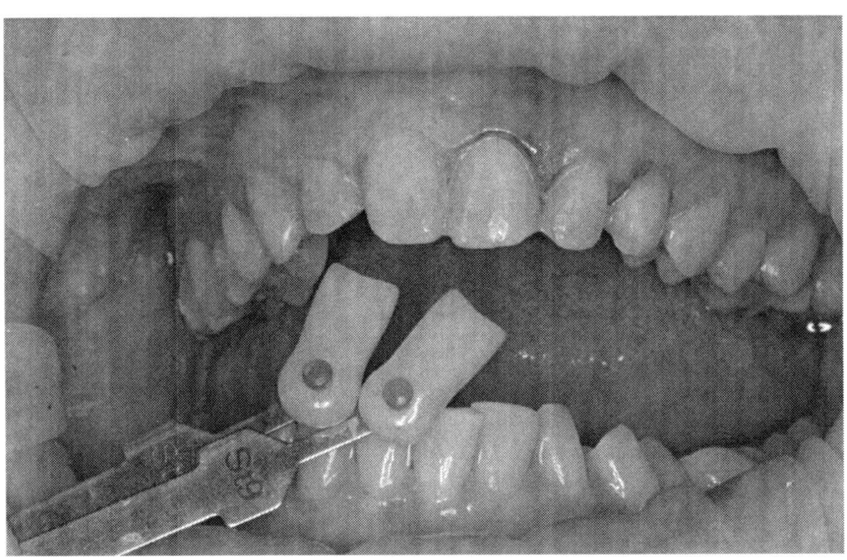

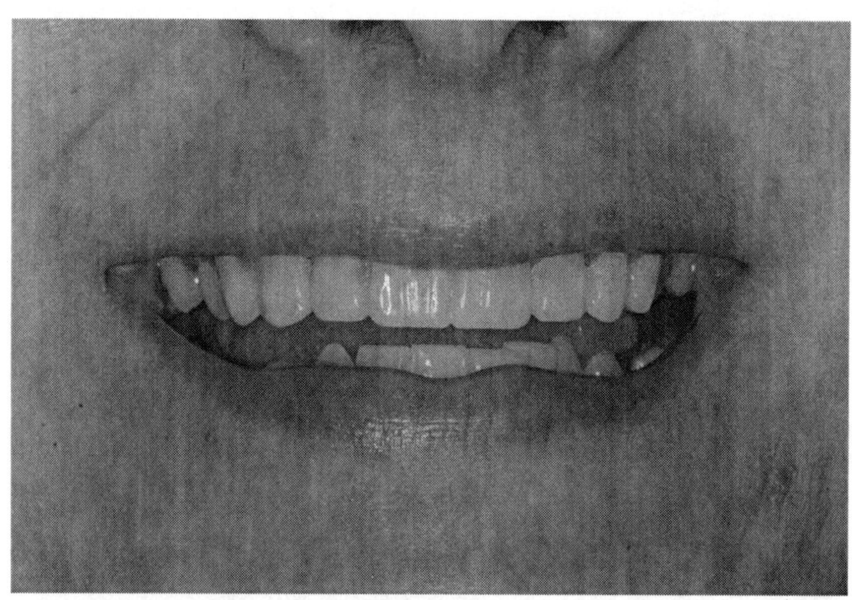

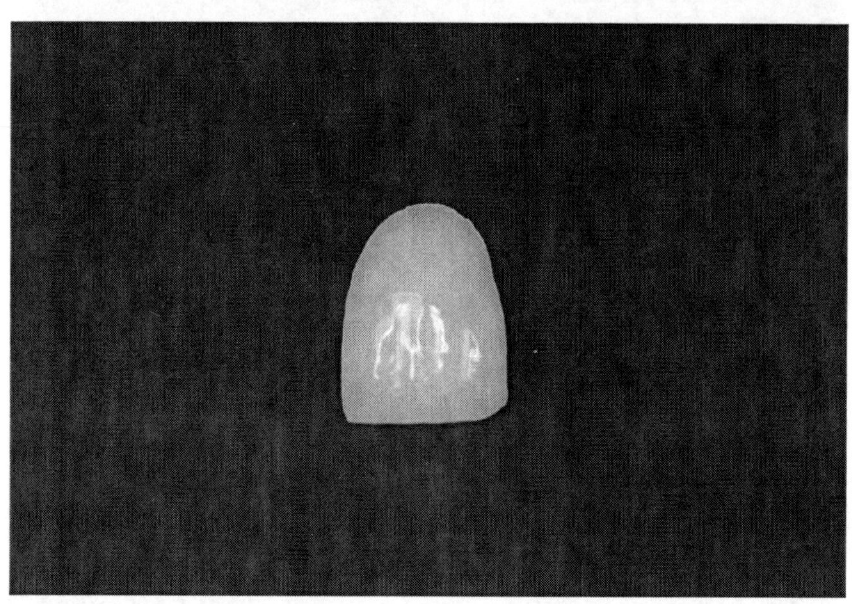

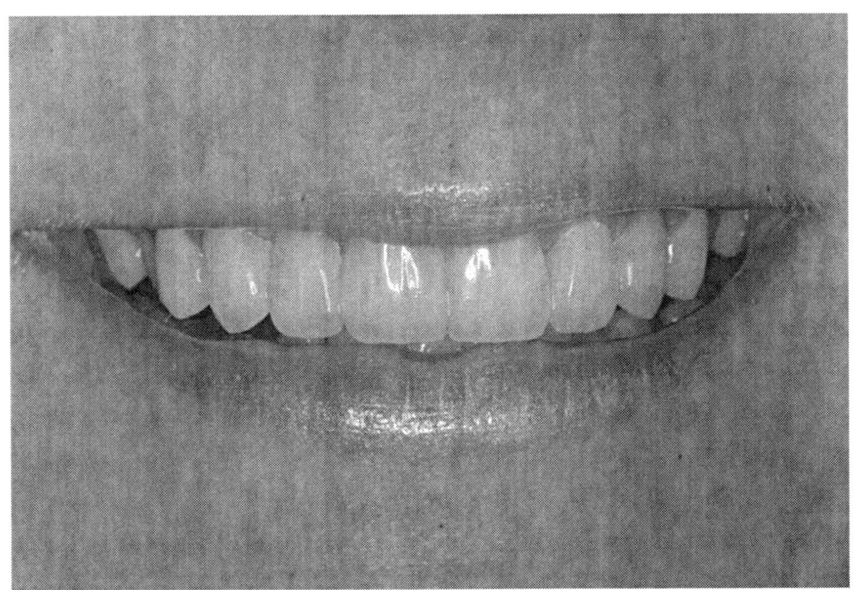

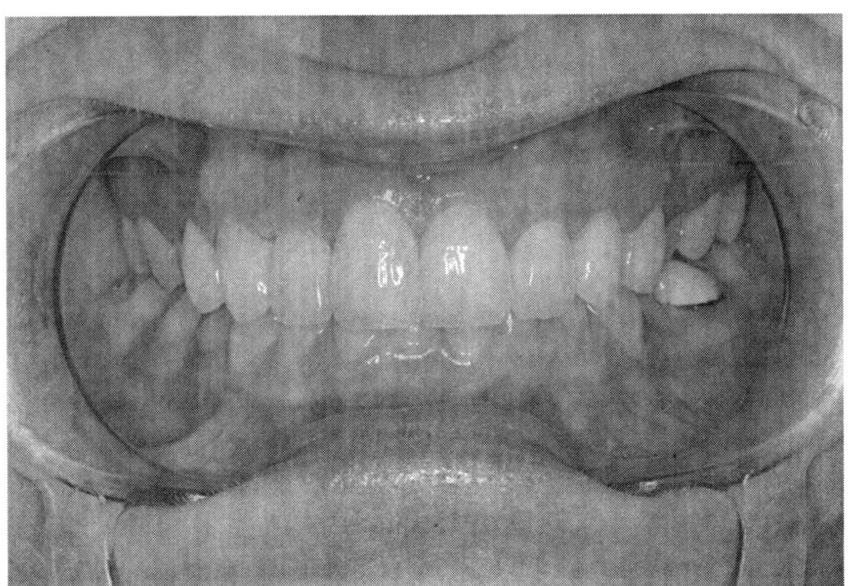

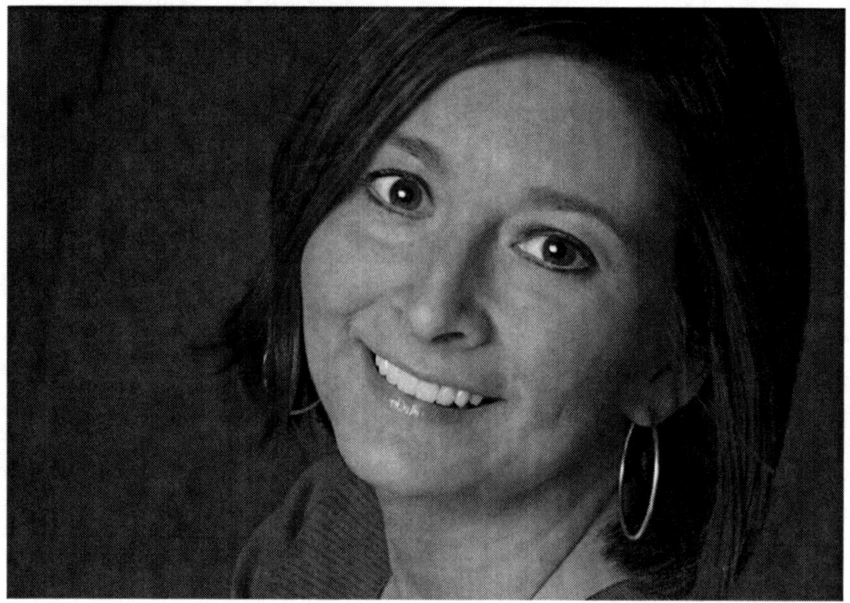

What are the pros and cons?

Every dental procedure comes with a list of pros and cons. Here are my thoughts on porcelain veneers:

- **Pros**: Porcelain veneers are very natural looking. They are permanently glued to your teeth so you don't have to take them in and out of your mouth under any circumstances. Porcelain veneers are also naturally stain-resistant, so unlike with your tooth's own enamel you won't have to worry about coffee, nicotine or tea stains. If properly cared for, veneers can last over a dozen years without complications, making them extremely durable and a good investment. Finally, veneers are one of the quickest options for transforming your smile.
- **Cons**: Because veneers oftentimes require removing the tooth's enamel, this procedure is irreversible. Once the enamel is removed, the tooth has been forever altered. Veneers are a costly investment compared to other smile makeover procedures. If you have a restricted budget, this may not be the option for you. If your veneers are not properly cared for, decay can form underneath them, they can chip, or even pop off of your teeth and then need them to be replaced at an additional fee.

How long does the procedure take?

Your porcelain veneers will require two visits after your initial consultation. Depending on the dental lab that your dentist uses, your veneers can be made in 5-14 business days. If you really need an instant smile makeover for a special occasion, some labs can even make them in just 2 business days for an additional fee!

How much will it cost?

Porcelain veneers will typically cost between $1,000 and $2,000 per tooth. The fees will vary depending on what region of the country you live as well as how skilled your cosmetic dentist is. Cheaper veneers are usually provided by dentists that are not using top notch dental labs/ceramists to make the veneers or dentists who are not as skilled.

Will insurance cover this procedure?

Porcelain veneers are considered a cosmetic procedure that is generally not covered by dental insurance. However, if your teeth have been affected by a medical circumstance such as taking certain antibiotics like tetracycline that stain your teeth or if you've suffered a severe accident, your dentist may be able to submit a letter with the history of your medical circumstance along with photos to attempt to get partial coverage.

How long will it last?

With normal wear and tear, your porcelain veneers can last between 15 to 20 years. Certain dental labs and cosmetic dentists stand behind their work and will offer a lifetime warranty. Ask your dentist if they offer a warranty to make sure that you get more bang for your buck.

A-List Advice:

Unsure if veneers are right for you? Ask your doctor for before and after pictures of their work. Make sure that you like the "veneer effect" before agreeing to the procedure.

Invisalign Clear Braces

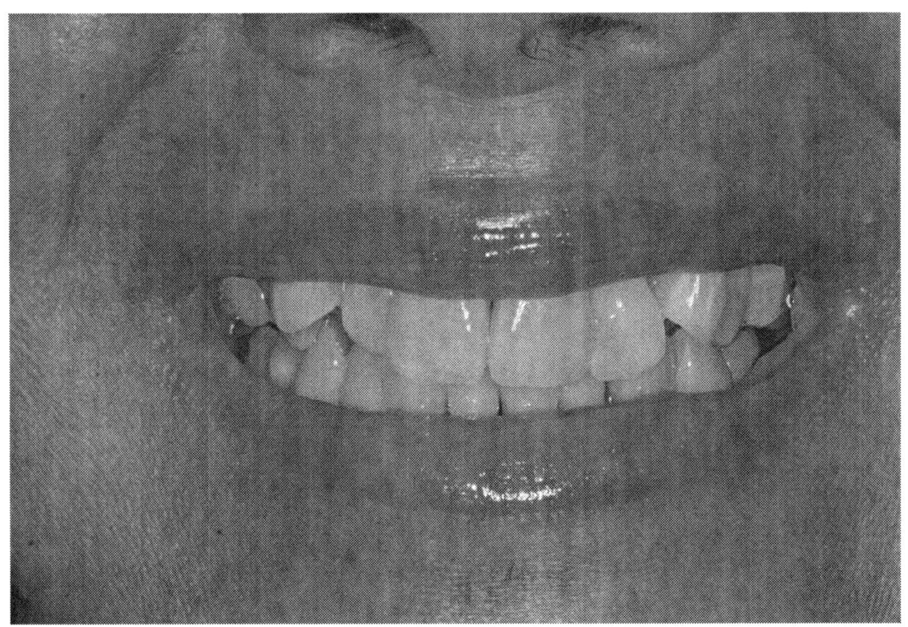

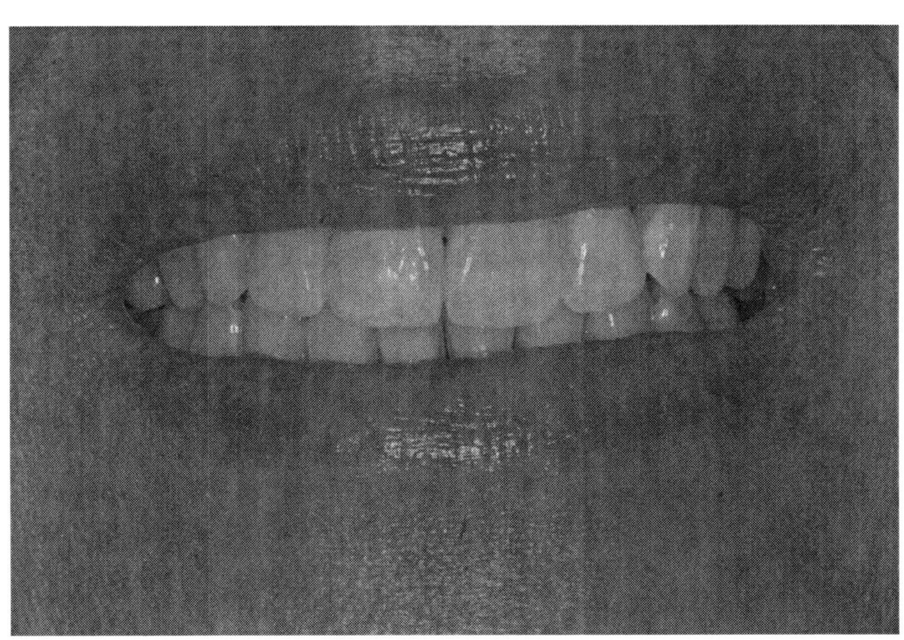

Back in the day, Kanye West had no choice but to wear simple wire braces, while pop star and fashion plate Gwen Stefani rocked her adult wire braces – proudly! As the "clear" alternative to wire braces, Invisalign is now the obvious choice for A-List stars seeking A-List smiles.

Vowing not to wed with crooked teeth, *Grey's Anatomy* and *27 Dresses* star Katherine Heigl opted for Invisalign to help straighten her teeth. Dr. Joyce Brothers, Cher, Venus Williams and even Tom Cruise have also worn braces as adults, capping their A-List status with A-List smiles. So if you want to have a stunning smile like Kanye, Katherine, Cher, Gwen Stefani or Tom Cruise, consider Invisalign.

Invisalign is an amazing new breakthrough technology that is quickly becoming one of the most popular ways to straighten misaligned teeth. Invisalign can be used to solve many orthodontic issues including rotated teeth, crowded teeth, widely spaced teeth, overbites, mild underbites and crossbites.

How does the procedure work?

An alternative to traditional braces, Invisalign works by using a series of custom-fabricated transparent molds called "aligners" that gradually shift your teeth into proper alignment. Because Invisalign requires no metal wires, no rubber bands, and no metal or white brackets, it's virtually undetectable, making it the treatment of choice among adult patients seeking orthodontic treatment.

During the first Invisalign visit, x-rays are taken, eight different photos are taken, putty moldings of your upper and lower teeth are made, and an imprint of your bite is made. Your Invisalign certified dentist will examine your teeth and fill out a prescription form to design your new smile. This prescription, along with the records, is sent to Invisalign to begin your smile design. Your records are scanned into a computer and Invisalign will begin to create a computerized digital image of your smile which is called a "Clin-check".

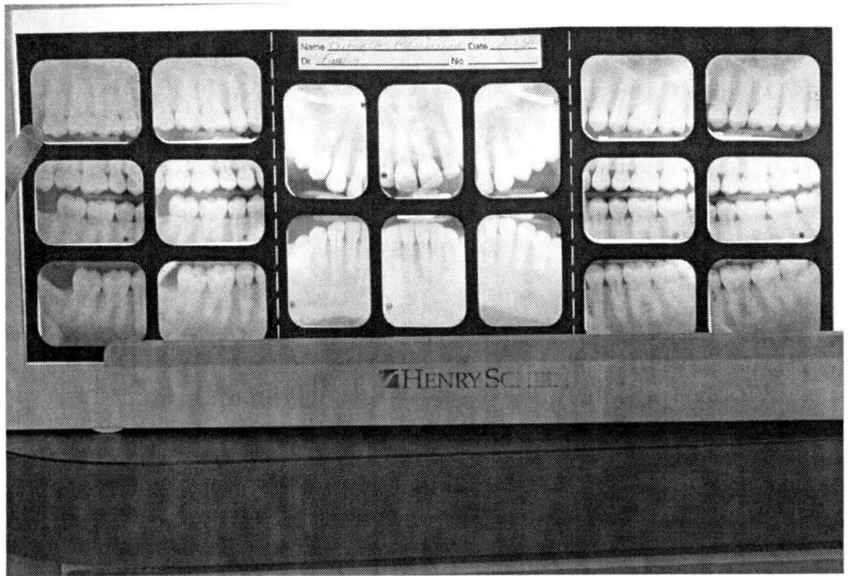

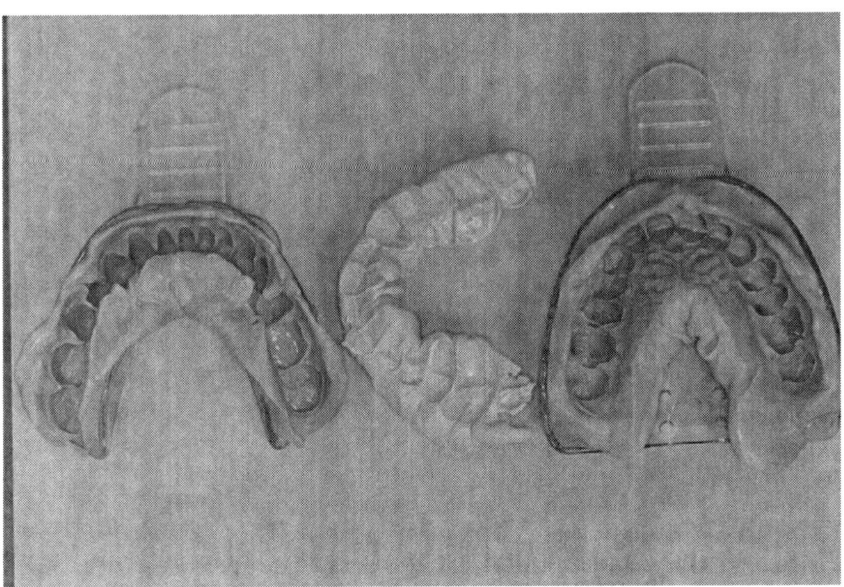

The second Invisalign visit is the viewing of the Clin-check. The Clin-check gives both the doctor and patient a step-by-step sneak preview of the predicted results of the Invisalign treatment. At this visit, the doctor is able to communicate how long you may have to wear the Invisalign aligners and any other details that will make the treatment a success. If you are happy with the predicted results, your dentist will authorize Invisalign to begin fabricating your aligners immediately. If you are not happy with the predicted results, your doctor can revise your prescription and Clin-check to improve your results.

The final Invisalign visit is the delivery and fitting of your aligners. Instructions are given for how to care for the aligners and you practice taking them in and out of your mouth before you are sent home with your cosmetic braces.

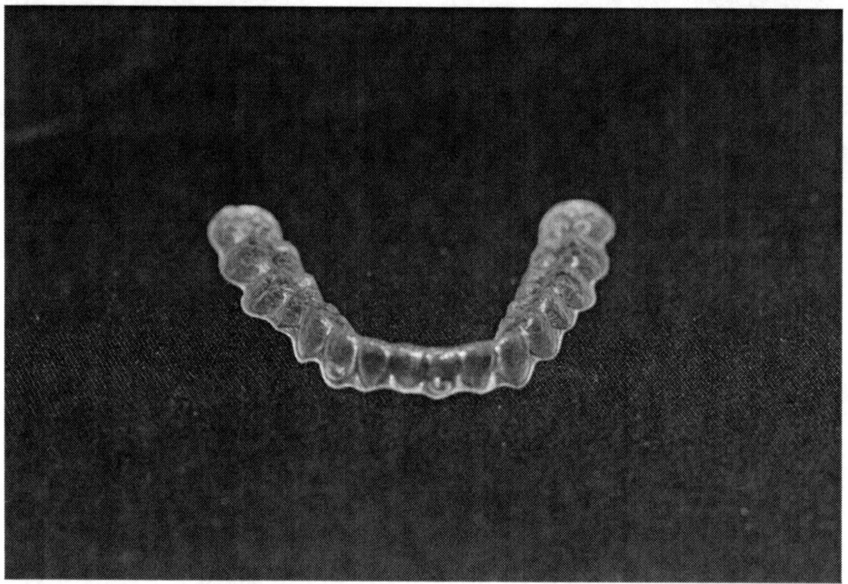

During the course of Invisalign treatment, patients wear anywhere from 12 to 22 different aligners (the number of aligners vary depending on each patient's specific needs). Patients wear the aligners during the day and through the night. The aligners are designed to be removed for eating, brushing, and flossing. Each aligner is worn for two weeks. Little by little, the teeth shift until the desired alignment is achieved.

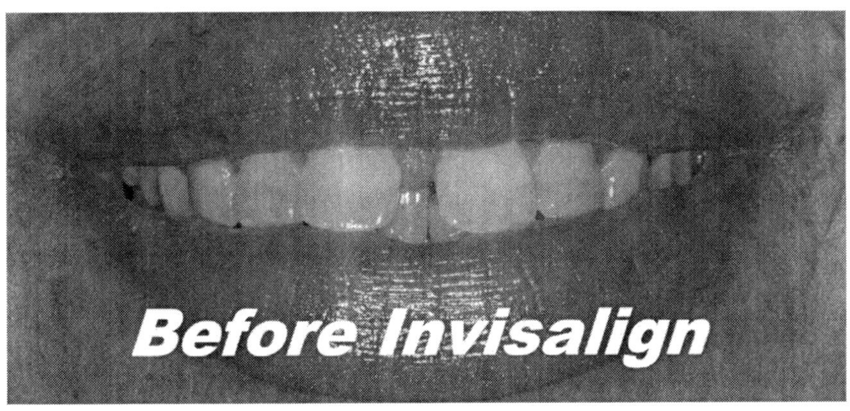
Before Invisalign

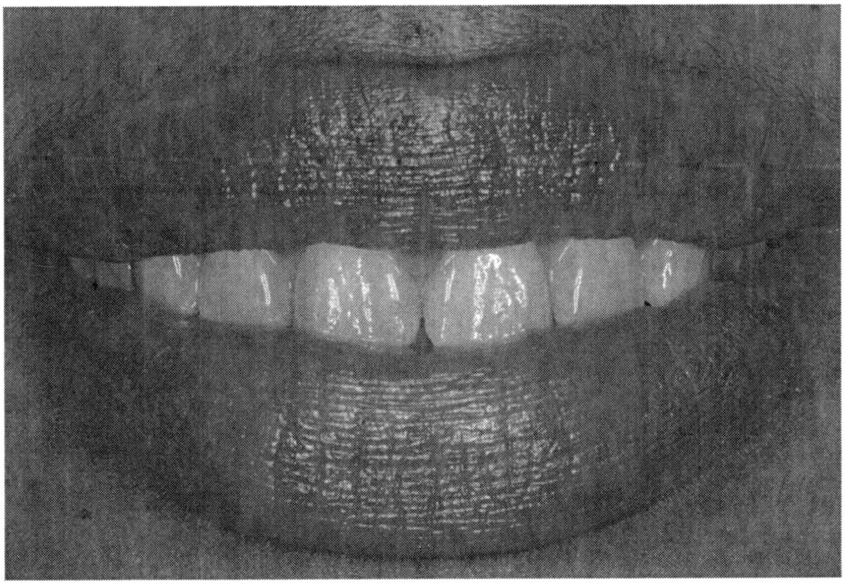

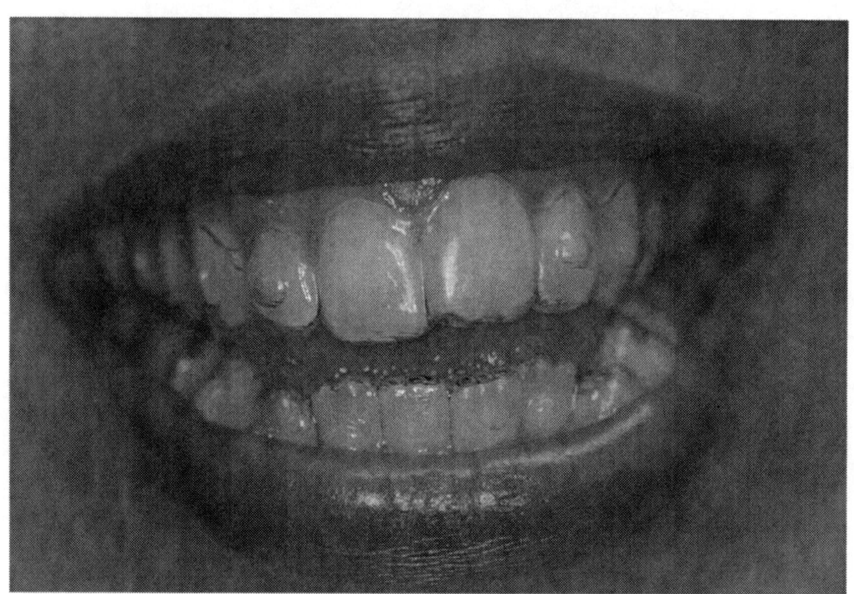

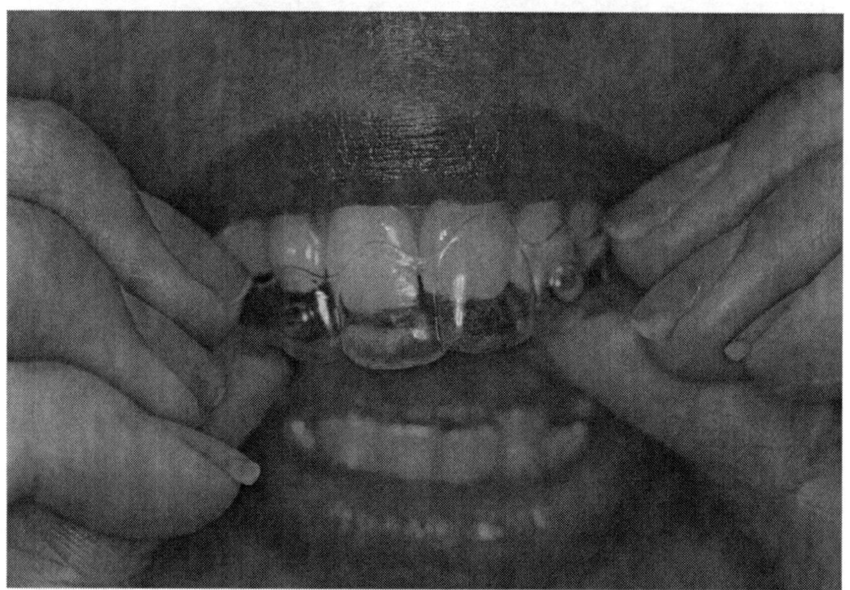

What are the pros and cons?

Every dental procedure comes with a list of pros and cons. Here are my thoughts concerning the pros and cons of the Invisalign treatment:

- **Pros**: These braces are practically invisible, so they are extremely attractive and hardly noticeable. They are perfect for the teenager or adult who wants to correct their smile without the embarrassment of wearing metal or white brackets on their teeth. Because the technology is so sophisticated and the computer-enhanced "aligners" so personalized, your braces are very flexible and comfortable to wear. They are also efficient at straightening your teeth in a much shorter time, drastically reducing the duration of metal braces, which is often up to two years. Invisalign is perfect for adults who once wore braces in their earlier years and have suffered a minor or even major relapse of the position of their teeth due to not wearing their retainer as prescribed. Most importantly, compared to the option of porcelain veneers, Invisalign is more affordable, reversible and the tooth's enamel remains preserved.
- **Cons**: Not every patient is a candidate for these clear braces. Patients with open bites, underbites, or that have teeth that are severely rotated or severely spaced may not qualify for Invisalign. Patients who are not responsible and compliant may not be suitable for Invisalign. After all, since the aligners are removable, the entire procedure depends on the patient being disciplined enough to wear them most of the day with the exception of taking them out to eat and taking them out to brush. If they are not worn as prescribed, they will not work.

How long does the procedure take?

From the initial visit, it takes two weeks to have a Clin-check made and then an additional two weeks from the approval of the Clin-check to have your aligners made (a total of a month to get the aligners). The average treatment time to correct mild dental problems is usually 6-11 months. More advanced dental cases will take 1-2 years.

How much will it cost?

Invisalign treatment will range depending on what region of the country you live in as well as if your Invisalign treatment is being performed by an orthodontist or an Invisalign certified cosmetic dentist. Average fees can range from $3,000 to $6,000.

Will insurance cover this procedure?

Invisalign treatment is an orthodontic service that can be submitted for payment or reimbursement by your insurance if your particular plan covers braces. Many insurance companies limit orthodontic benefits to patients who are 19 years old or younger. However, some plans do extend benefits to adult patients. If you are considering braces, contact your dental insurance company to see if they offer benefits for this service.

How long will it last?

Invisalign results can last forever if a retainer is worn daily for a lifetime. I've seen patients wear their retainer religiously for a couple of years and then stop, assuming that it would be okay, only to discover that their teeth slowly but surely began to go back to their original position. Many of my patients are choosing to permanently retain their teeth with a non-visible wire that is placed on the back of the teeth so that the teeth are locked and can't move.

A-List Advice:

Although Invisalign invisible braces may be alluring, discuss the specifics of your situation with your dentist. If traditional braces work better, use them!

ZOOM! Teeth Whitening

Virtually all celebs whiten their teeth. In fact, teeth whitening is the #1 most requested procedure from my celeb clients. Some celebs are even obsessed with whitening, like Omarosa from *The Apprentice* who recently mentioned on the Discovery Health show *Plastic Surgery: Before and After* that she "can't get enough" of it.

When I was the spokesperson for Aquafresh, I was able to give tons of A-list stars teeth whitening products to keep their smiles bright. Actress America Ferrera of *Ugly Betty* even had her white smile insured for 1 million dollars! Teeth whitening is the most popular and cost effective procedures that can give you an instant A-List smile like the stars.

Teeth whitening is also one of the quickest, most popular and non-invasive ways to improve the appearance of your smile. If your teeth are not their brightest due to beverage stains, antibiotic use or simply the effects of time, teeth whitening may be the solution. Teeth whitening technology makes it easy for you to safely and effectively brighten your teeth, eliminating discolorations and enhancing your overall appearance.

To dramatically whiten your teeth, most dental experts now use ZOOM!, one of the leading teeth whitening systems available. With the ZOOM! gel and light-activated whitening system, we can actually lighten the color of your teeth an average of eight shades in just under an hour.

How does the procedure work?

To determine if you are a candidate for teeth whitening, your dentist will examine the health of your teeth and gums, the color of your teeth and look for any potential roadblocks that may affect the outcome of the whitening results such as the presence of visible bondings or crowns on your front teeth that will not lighten during the whitening procedure. If there are stains, plaque or tartar on your teeth, you may be required to have a professional teeth cleaning prior to your whitening treatment. If there are extremely large cavities present, you may be required to repair them first before cosmetically enhancing your smile with teeth whitening to avoid complications.

To begin the procedure, your dentist will take "before" photos that will be used to later compare the initial color of your teeth to the final color after whitening.

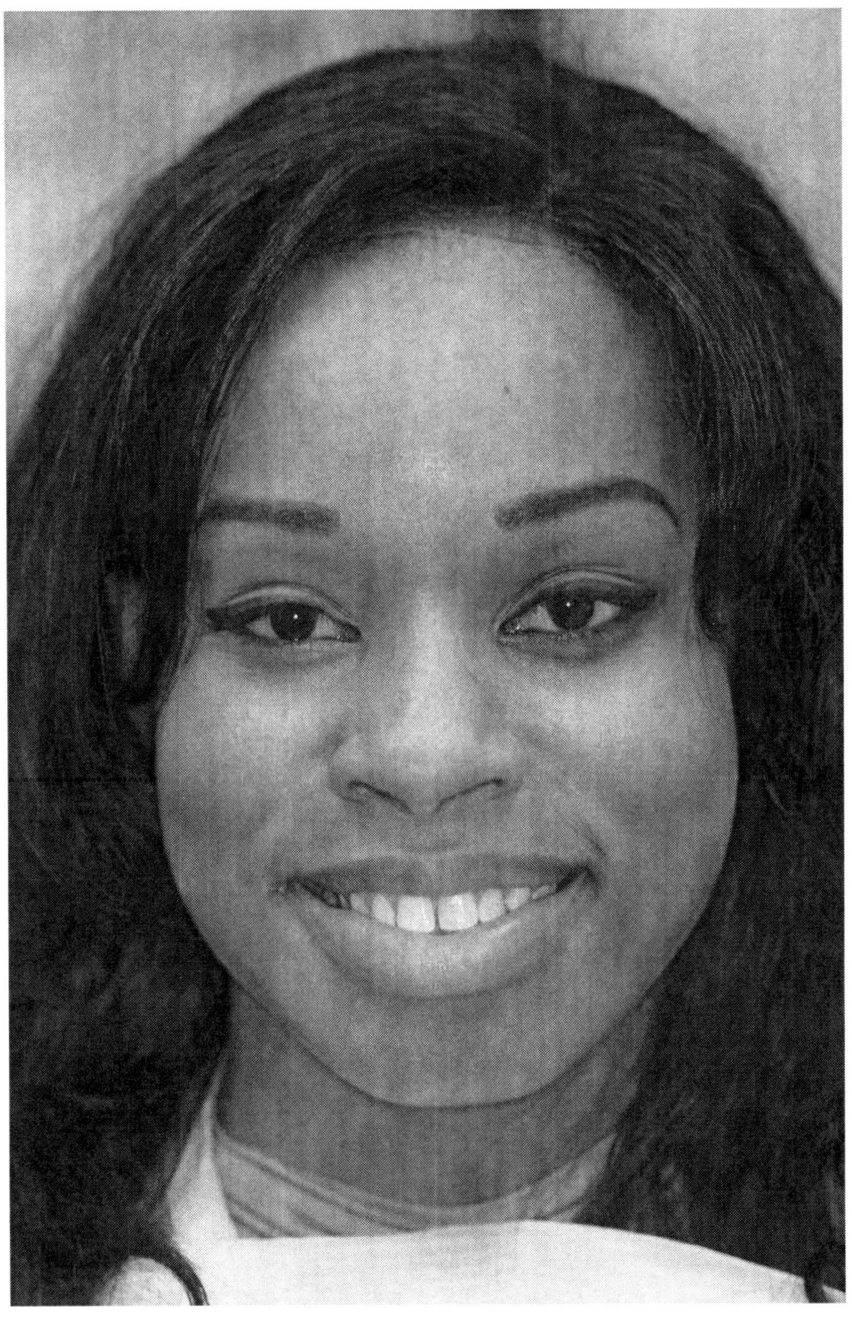

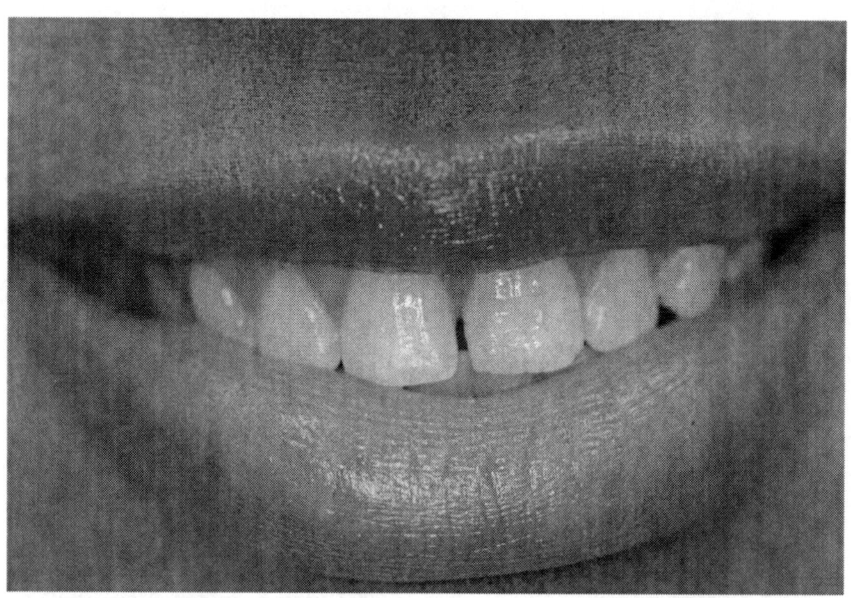

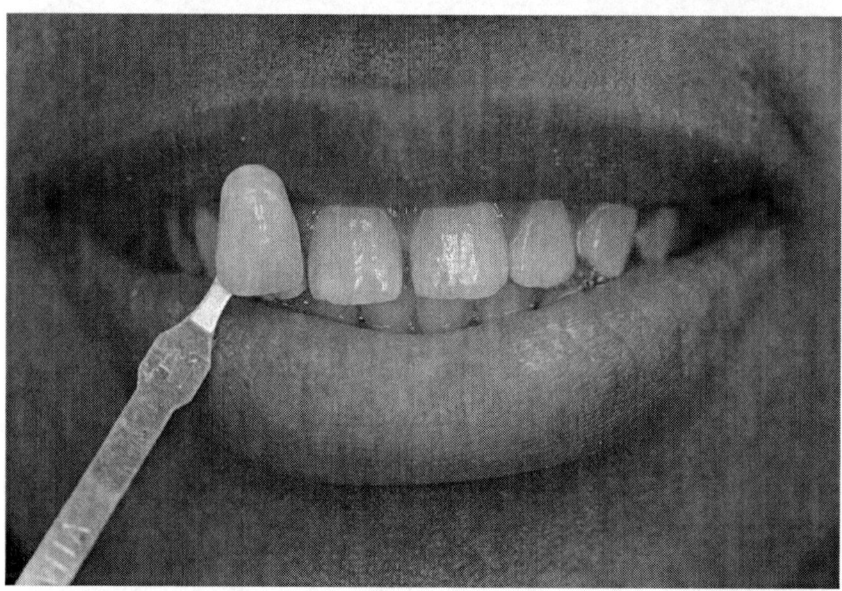

Next, your dentist will begin protecting your cheeks, lips and gums with barrier materials so that only your teeth are exposed.

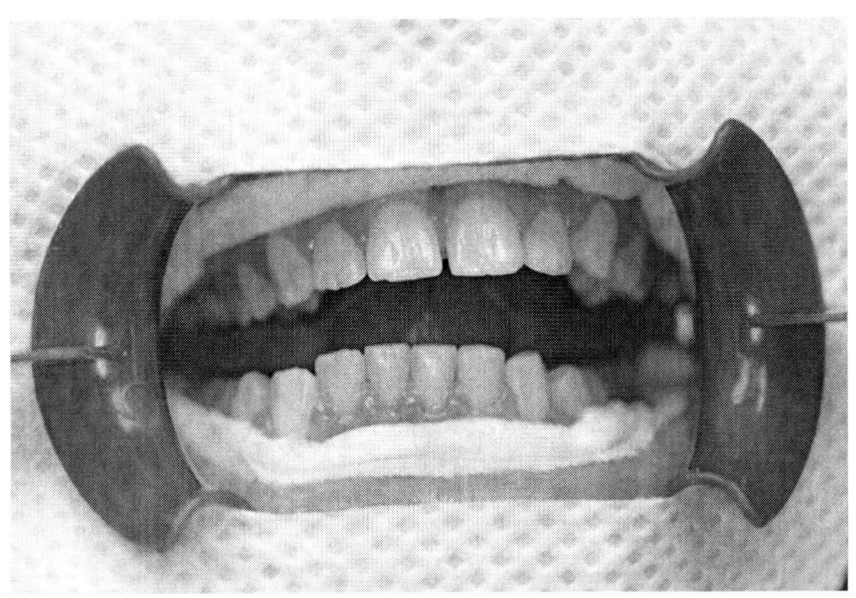

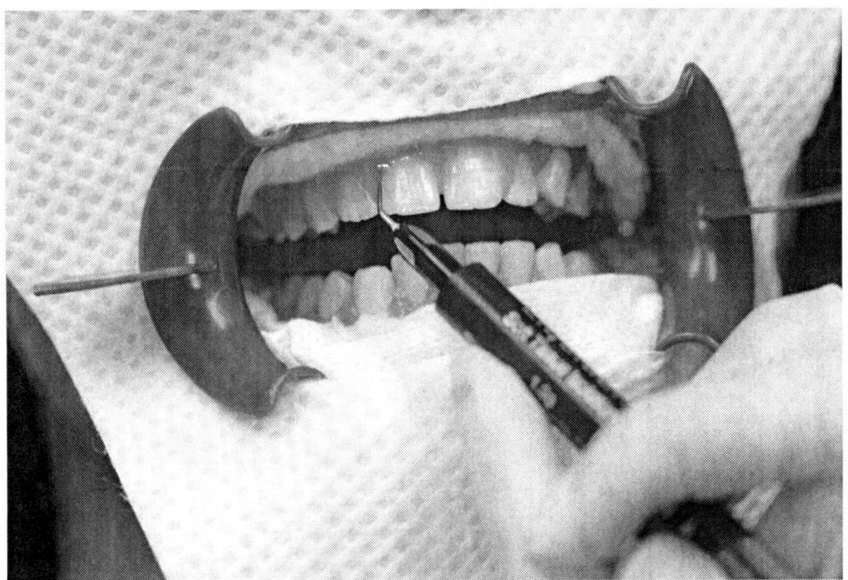

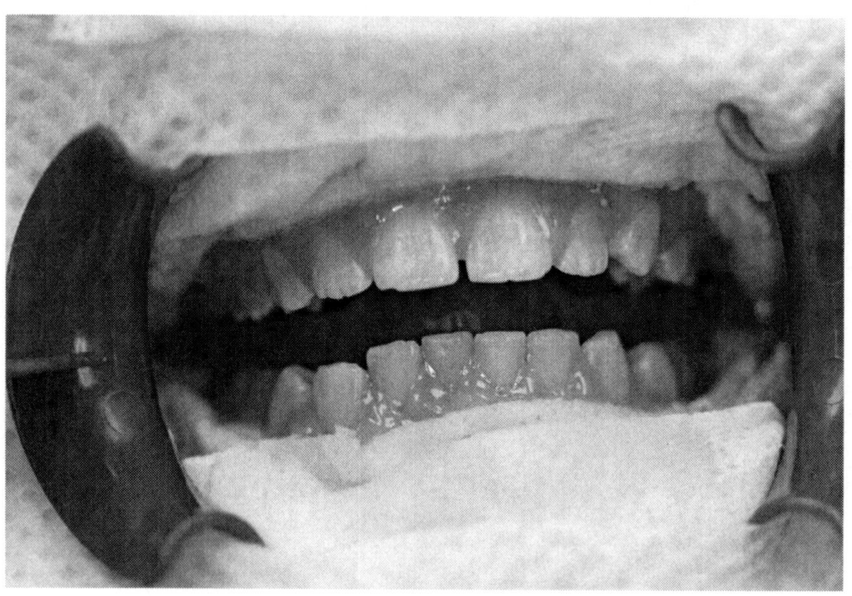

The ZOOM! peroxide teeth whitening gel is applied directly to the teeth and activated by the ZOOM! whitening lamp.

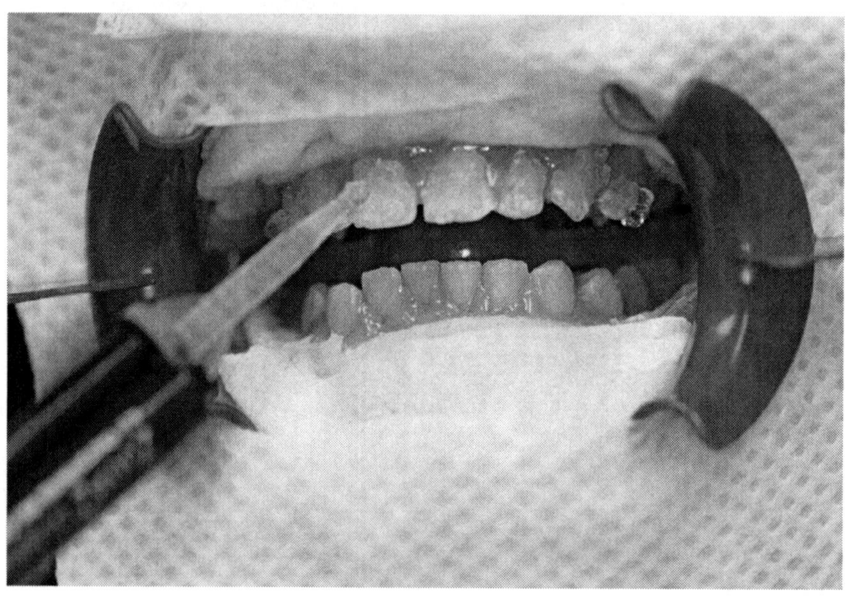

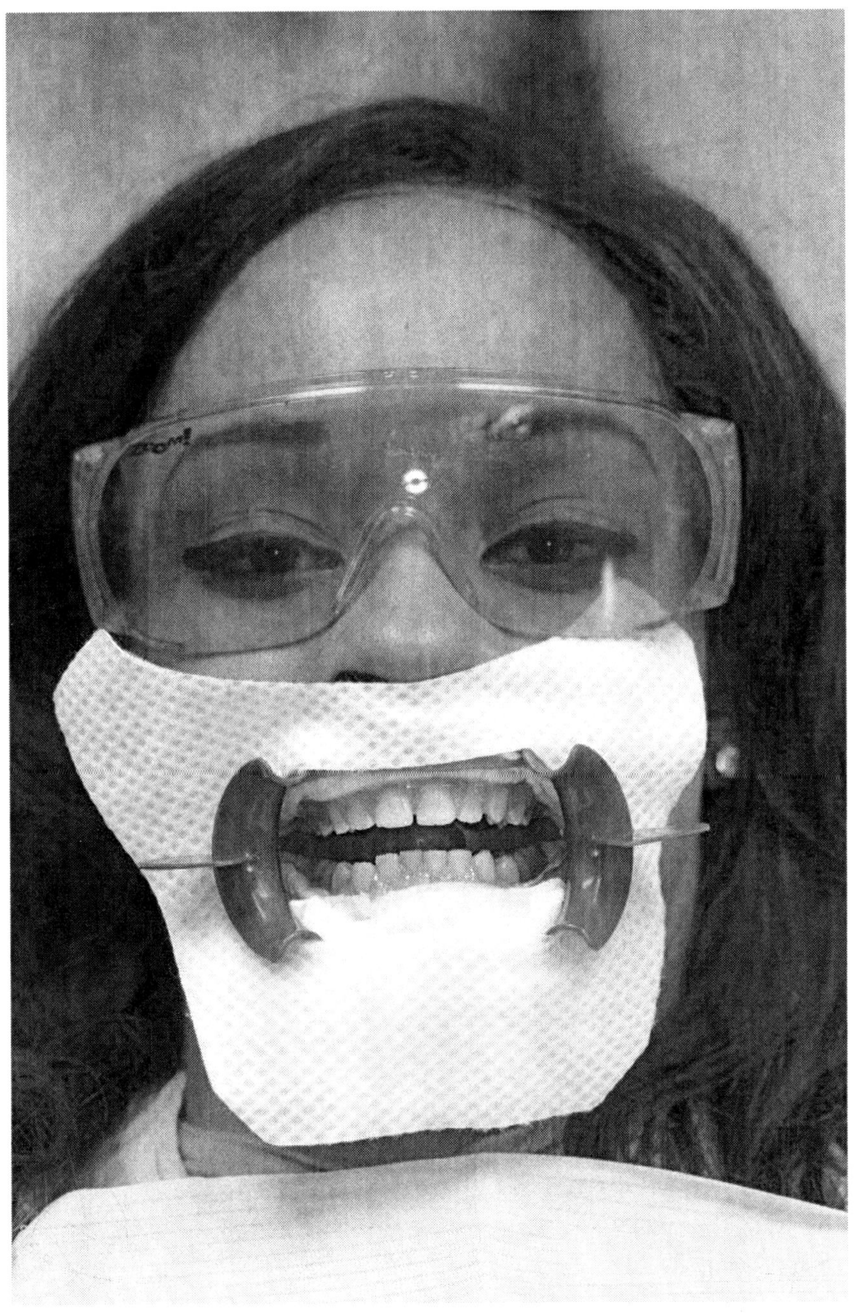

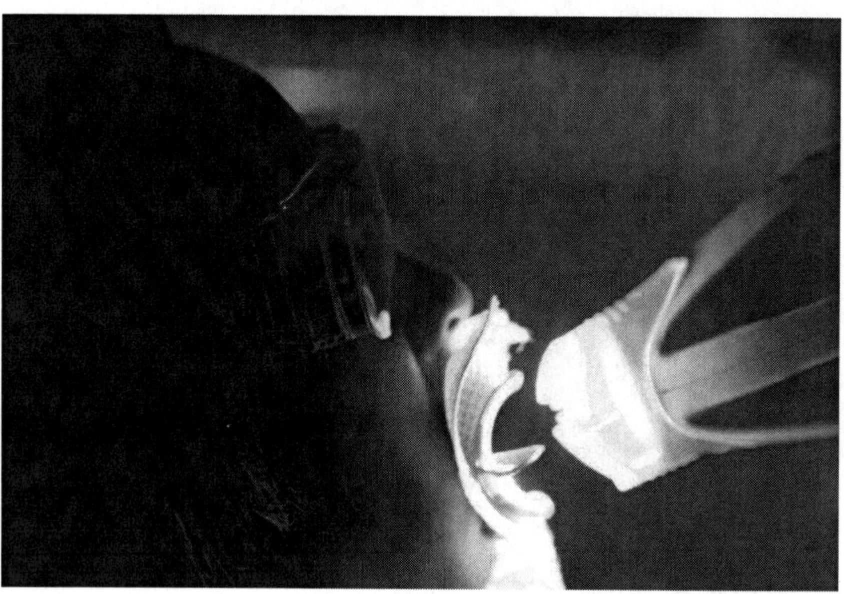

The gel is applied to the teeth 4 times for 15 minutes each session to total 1 hour. While you relax each 15 minute session, many dentists even let you view a movie on a monitor, or listen to music on headsets. In the meantime, the peroxide teeth whitening gel is foaming and working in the layer below the tooth's enamel to get them their whitest. After the 4th session, your dentist will take "after" photos to show you just how much whiter your teeth are following treatment. Our patients are always thrilled with the results.

What are the pros and cons?

Every dental procedure comes with a list of pros and cons. Here are my thoughts concerning the pros and cons of the ZOOM! whitening process:

- **Pros**: The ZOOM! whitening gel is one of the strongest on the market and yields some of the best whitening results possible. It's much more effective than any over the counter whitening system that is on the shelves of your local pharmacy or grocery store. Just one hour out of your day is all it takes for bright, white results.

- **Cons**: The actual results of teeth whitening are completely unpredictable. The whitening procedure does not always yield the results that the dentist predicts before the procedure. The teeth whitening procedure does not work effectively on all stains and discolorations. Teeth that have grey or brown tones do not respond to the whitening gel as well as teeth that have yellow tones. If whitening does not yield the results that you desire, you may have to consider porcelain veneers to mask your discoloration. Like all whitening products there are possible side effects that can occur during and after the whitening treatment. The most common side effect is teeth sensitivity. Since the whitening gel works on the inside layer of the teeth where the nerve is located, tooth sensitivity can occur. If it does occur, it usually will not last more than 24 hours. The second common side effect is irritation of the gums and other tissues surrounding the teeth. If the peroxide gel makes contact with the gums, the gum tissue can temporarily turn white (lasting only for about 1 hour). Your whitening specialist can prevent this by protecting your gums with barrier material. Despite these possible side effects, professional teeth whitening remains a safe procedure that can make a huge difference in your appearance.

How much will it cost?

ZOOM! whitening treatment will range depending on what region of the country you live and the experience of your dental provider. ZOOM! can range between $350 to $800 per procedure.

Will insurance cover this procedure?

Teeth whitening is considered a cosmetic procedure that is generally not covered by dental insurance. However, if your teeth have been affected by a medical circumstance such as taking certain antibiotics like tetracycline that stain your teeth, your dentist may be able to submit a letter with the history of your medical circumstance along with photos to attempt to get partial coverage.

How long will it last?

Whitening your teeth is similar to dying your hair; over time the procedure needs to be touched up to keep it fresh. If regular maintenance isn't performed, the whitening procedure will need to be redone sooner than necessary. ZOOM! in-office whitening results can last up to two years by visiting your dentist at least twice a year for a professional teeth cleaning to remove any stains, plaque or tartar that may have accumulated.

If you follow a routine dental protocol at home of brushing with a soft or preferably a powerful electric toothbrush, use a baking soda formula toothpaste to act as an abrasive to minimize the stains, and monitor your consumption of foods and beverages that can stain your teeth, your teeth will remain white longer. Between ZOOM! whitening sessions, you can also maintain optimal whiteness by using take home whitening trays and gel that your dentist can provide or use the popular over the counter whitening strips and trays that are found in your local stores.

> **A-List Advice:**
>
> *Use the opportunity of a ZOOM! whitening process to change the habits that led to your stained teeth in the first place. If you smoke, try to quit. If you drink a lot of coffee and tea, cut down and begin using a straw to decrease staining in the future.*

Snap-On Smile

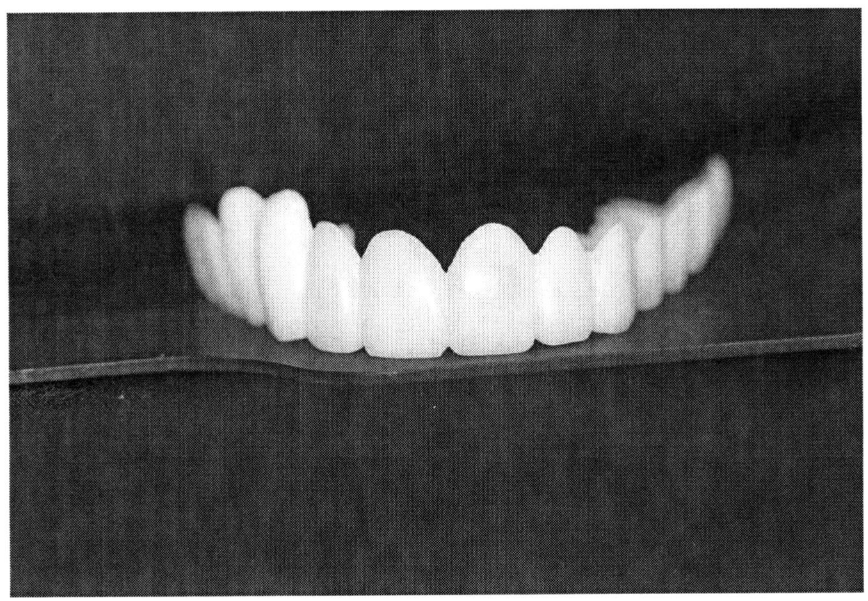

The Snap-On Smile is an appliance that can give you an A-List Smile without having an A-list budget. Your favorite A-Lister will not likely be sporting one since they usually prefer to invest in the more permanent option of veneers to enhance their smile, but the Snap-On Smile is a perfect start for someone who wants to look good and is on a budget.

The Snap-On Smile created by Dr. Marc Liechtung is an exciting, state-of-the-art cosmetic dental appliance that gives patients many of the benefits of cosmetic dentistry without the cost or commitment of more intensive, often irreversible procedures.

If you have misaligned teeth, missing teeth or poor caps and veneers – or you would simply like to preview what permanent cosmetic dentistry can do for you – many dental experts now offer Snap-On Smile at their dental practices as an easy and affordable solution.

How does the procedure work?

First, your dentist makes a putty molding of your existing teeth to replicate the existing smile. Second, your dentist will give you the opportunity to choose the preferred shape and color of your Snap-On. From the "smile-style" book, patients can choose from 19 color shades and over 18 shapes and teeth arrangements. The Snap-On accessory can even be modeled after your favorite celebrity's smile! You can pick the Julia Roberts, Denzel, or the most popular request… the Halle Berry. Third, your case is sent to the Snap-On laboratory for custom fabrication and within 10-14 days, your beautiful Snap-on Smile is ready.

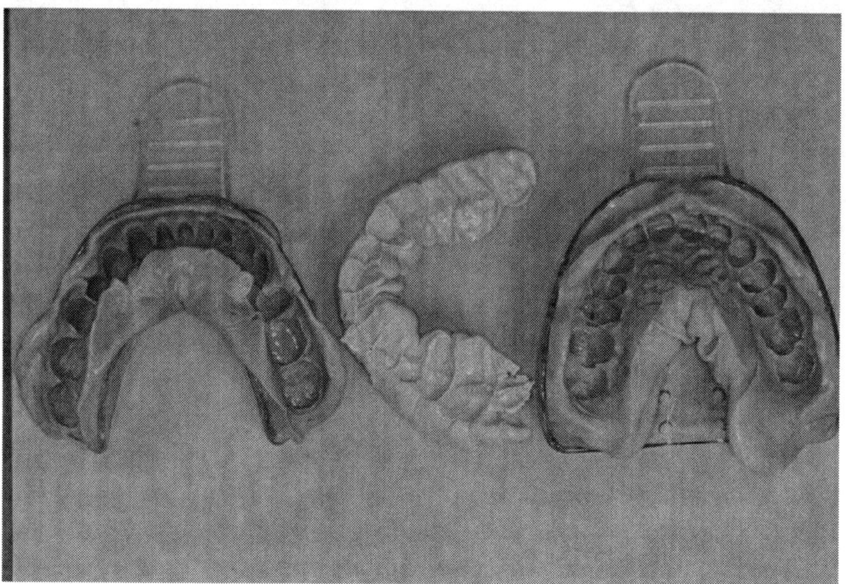

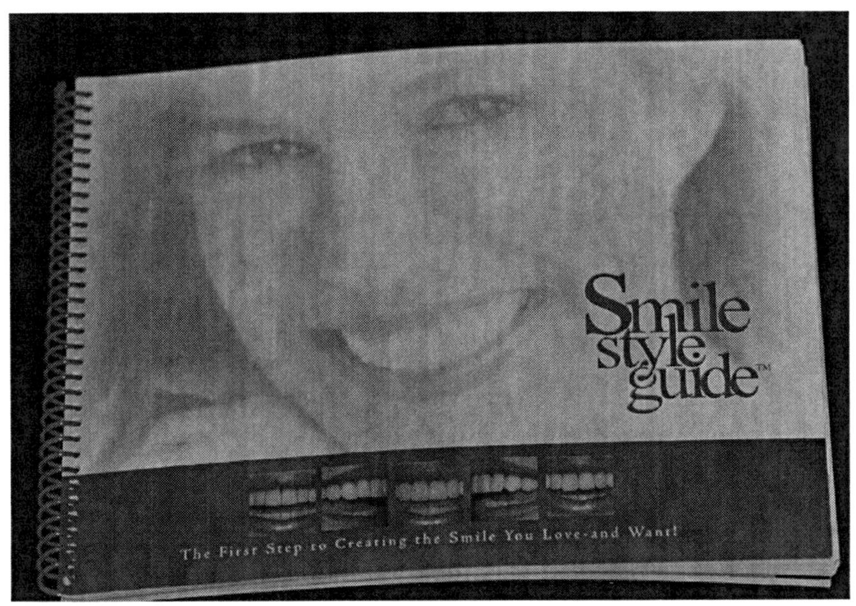
Smile
style
guide™
The First Step to Creating the Smile You Love–and Want!

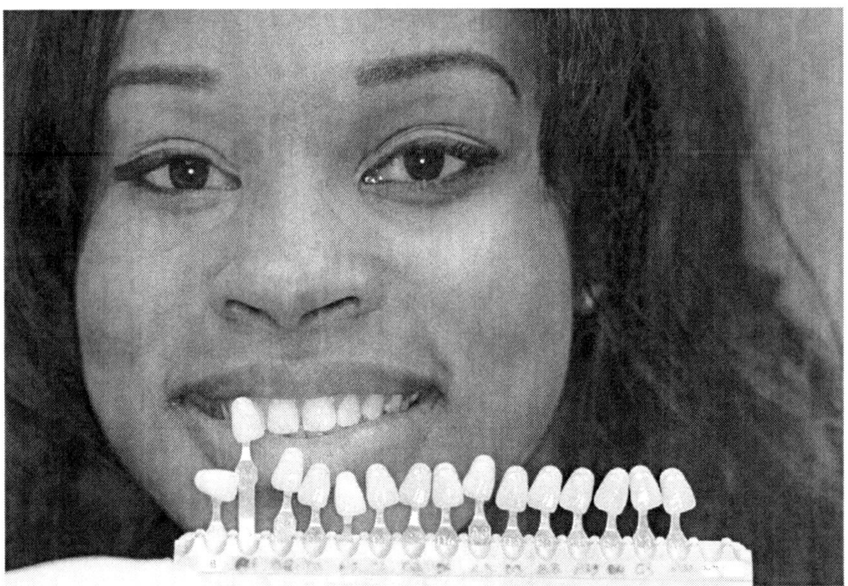

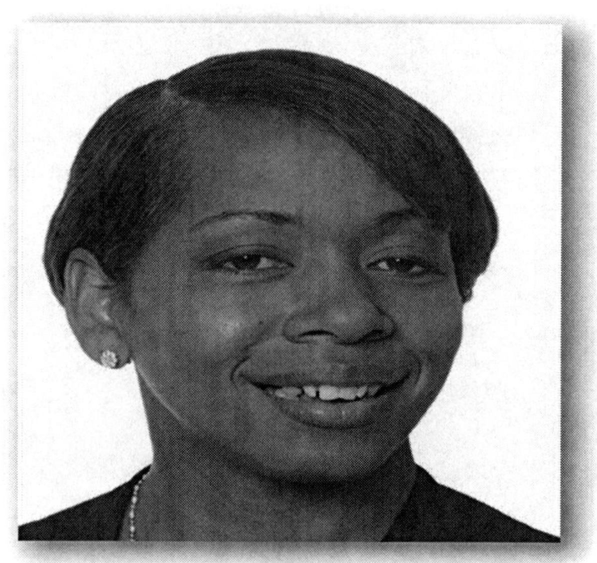

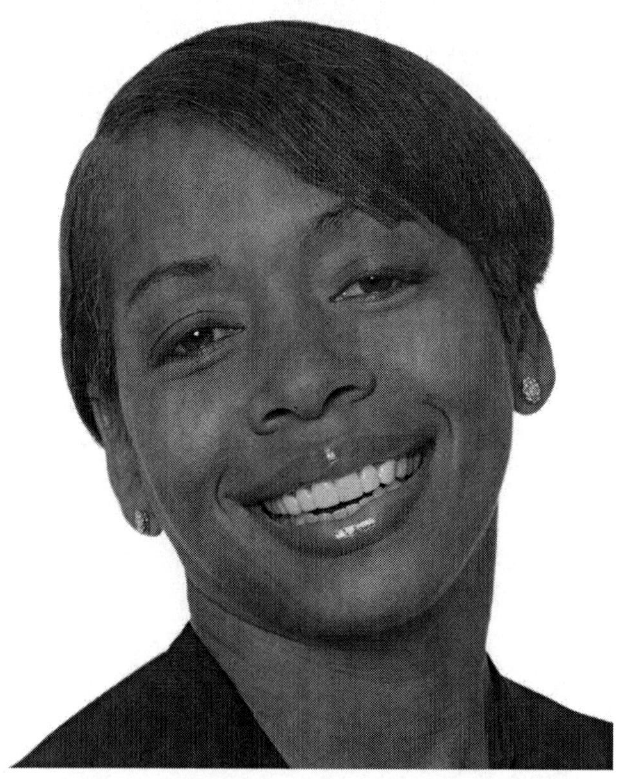

The perfect candidate for the Snap-On Smile may be a bride-to-be or teen with limited funds who is taking pictures in a few weeks. Aspiring actors, singers, or models can use the Snap-On for headshots or to nail the job. Quite frankly, any patient who is looking for an affordable cosmetic alternative to permanent dental work such as veneers can benefit from this amazing accessory. You simply "snap on" the appliance and go confidently about your day with your beautiful new A-List Smile.

To remove the Snap-On Smile appliance, gently rock it from side to side until it loosens, and then pull it out. Your Snap-On Smile appliance can be maintained with normal hygiene and overnight soaking. Your dental expert will walk you through every step of the insertion and maintenance process so that you always feel comfortable and confident with your beautiful new smile.

What are the pros and cons?

Every dental procedure comes with a list of pros and cons. Here are my thoughts concerning the pros and cons of the Snap-On Smile:

- **Pros**: The beauty of this procedure is there are no shots and no changes to your natural tooth structure with drilling is needed. Have a fear of the dentist but want a beautiful smile? The Snap-On Smile is an easy, pain free option to enhance your smile. The Snap-On Smile is a reversible procedure that does not require the use of adhesive; it's completely removable when need be. Your Snap-On Smile appliance can even be worn while you eat and drink. Because of its highly specialized, elastic material, the Snap-On Smile appliance adapts snuggly to your teeth. As a result, there's never any uncomfortable brittleness, and you don't have to worry about the appliance cracking when you put it on. It's perfect for teens and adults of all ages, especially baby boomers who are interested in rejuvenating their smiles without much invasion of their natural teeth.
- **Cons**: While many patients have had success with the Snap-On

Smile, others have found better success with veneers, bridges and braces because the results are more permanent and more natural looking.

How much will it cost?

The estimated cost for your Snap-On Smile ranges from $1,000-$2,000 for each arch of the mouth. This fee is non-refundable. Compare this to the price of permanent porcelain veneers, which can range from $1,000-$2,000 per tooth and the Snap-On Smile is definitely something to smile about.

Will insurance cover this procedure?

The Snap-On Smile is generally considered a cosmetic procedure that is not covered by dental insurance. However, if you are missing teeth and if your plan offers benefits for major services such as teeth replacements, they *may* cover your Snap-On Smile.

If you want to be certain of the benefits offered by your plan before starting your work, your dentist may be willing to submit a letter with x-rays to your insurance company to get a pre-authorization of the procedure with fees that they will pay as well as fees that will be due by you.

How long will it last?

Your Snap-On Smile can last an average of 3-5 years, the same as any removable partial denture or appliance, i.e. night guards, etc. We do advise that proper care is needed. Although this procedure is non-refundable, it does come with a 60 day warranty.

A-List Advice:

The Snap-On Smile® is one of the secret weapons that many of my nervous patients choose to enhance their smiles. If you've been putting off your smile makeover due to fear, you may want to consider this pain free smile makeover technique.

Tooth-colored Fillings:
Composite Resin and Inlays

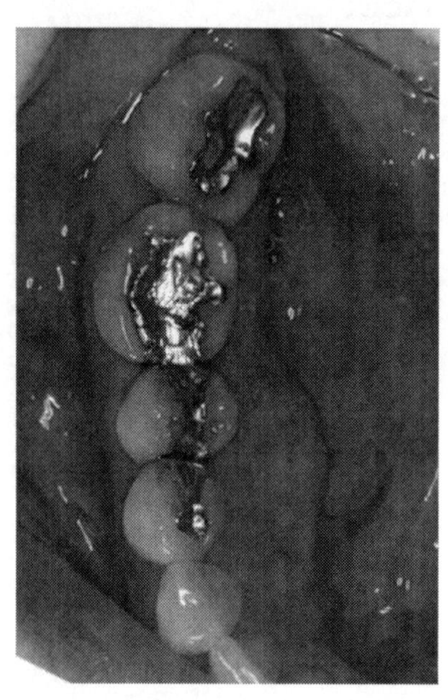

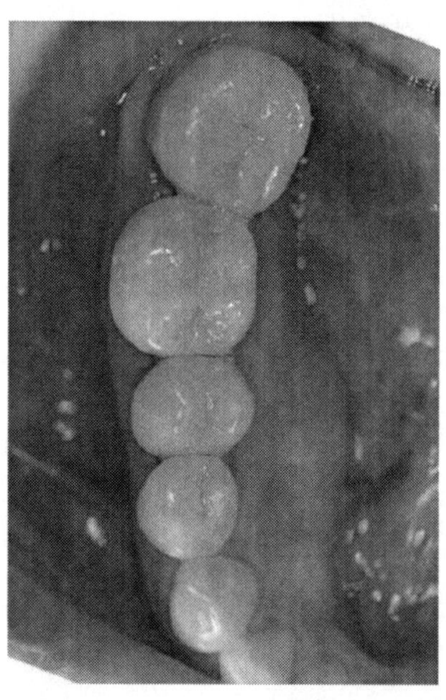

Many celebs want to hide those old, unsightly silver fillings. One popular New York on-air personality that is big on smiles had me remove every single silver filling and replace them with the porcelain fillings – the result was amazing! The number one question that celebs ask me is, "Is it safe to remove the silver?"

In most instances, the answer is, "Yes." Before changing the silver, it's important that your dentist review your most current set of x-rays to determine how deep your existing silver filling is. The deeper the filling is, the closer to the nerve it may be. The closer the filling is to the nerve, the greater chances of having prolonged tooth sensitivity, which could potentially lead to a root canal.

So have your dentist tell you if you are a candidate for changing your silver fillings and your risk level of having sensitivity. Changing your silver fillings is another procedure that can give you an instant A-List Smile like the stars.

Dentistry has come a long way since the time when metal amalgam fillings were the norm. Advanced materials give today's dental professionals more freedom to create natural-looking fillings that are both aesthetically and structurally superior to their predecessors.

Advances in modern dental materials have enabled doctors to treat teeth that are decayed, damaged or worn with tooth-colored fillings. Your dental expert can repair teeth and replace old fillings using natural-looking porcelain or plastic "composite resin" materials that are carefully matched to the color of your existing teeth. Porcelain tooth-colored fillings which are called "inlays" provide the same protection as silver while remaining virtually invisible and are now considered to be "state-of the-art" and the "new standard of care" in dentistry.

How does the procedure work?

Depending on the depth of the cavity or chip, numbing may or may not be needed. The necessary drilling is performed to remove the decay or existing silver filling or reshape the chipped tooth in preparation for your tooth colored filling. If you and your dentist choose to use the stronger porcelain "inlay" to fill the tooth, a molding is taken of the tooth, it is sent to the porcelain lab and a temporary filling is placed in the tooth to be worn as your inlay is being made.

A second visit is needed to permanently place the filling. All tooth colored fillings are adhered to the tooth structure by way of bonding. First, A mild acid is placed on the tooth to "open the pores" of the outer and inner tooth structure. Next, the dentist will place a liquid adhesive in the tooth that acts as a "glue" to hold and eventually lock the filling material inside the pores of the tooth.

The filling is then secured and locked with an UV light. If you and your dentist choose to use the plastic composite resin to fill the tooth, your dentist will have the material in his or her office and will select and place the color material that matches your tooth the best. Once your filling is placed, it is smoothed and shaped properly as well as polished to feel as normal as your original tooth felt.

What are the pros and cons?

Every dental procedure comes with a list of pros and cons. Here are my thoughts concerning the pros and cons of dental fillings:

- **Pros**: Tooth-colored fillings are as strong as metal fillings. They can even be used to repair back teeth, where pressure from chewing is greatest. Tooth-colored fillings also support the remaining tooth structure, helping to prevent breaks and cracks and insulating the tooth from extreme temperature changes. Additionally, because they contain no mercury, tooth-colored fillings eliminate the health risks associated with metal fillings.
- **Cons**: Because tooth-colored fillings require a more time-intensive procedure to apply, they can be slightly more costly then traditional metal fillings. If you choose the stronger porcelain inlay as your material, it requires an extra visit to complete the procedure. If you select the plastic composite resin as your material, your dentist has to hand sculpt your filling, which leaves room for errors in placement. Tooth colored fillings can pick up stains over time and lose their natural luster if they are not cared for properly.

How much will it cost?

Despite their many added benefits to metal fillings, tooth-colored, resin-based fillings are only moderately more expensive than the traditional variety, costing between $150 to $200 per filling.

Will insurance cover this procedure?

Tooth colored fillings placed on the back molar teeth are generally not fully covered by dental insurance. The rules for each insurance plan may differ depending on the benefits package that you choose. Typically, insurance companies do what's called a "downgrade" where they will give the patient the money for a silver filling and then have the patient pay the difference between the cost of the white filling and silver filling.

If your plan offers benefits for basic or major services such as plastic composite resin fillings or porcelain inlays, then they may cover your tooth colored filling. If you want to be certain of the benefits offered by your plan before starting your work, your dentist may be willing to submit a letter with x-rays to your insurance to get a pre-authorization of the procedure with fees that they will pay as well as fees that you will need to cover.

How long will it last?

The type of material used for your tooth-colored fillings will determine life expectancy. Porcelain inlays can last approximately 10 or more years. Plastic composite resins are expected to last an average of 3-5 years.

A-List Advice:

Be proactive about dental health now, while you are still in the planning stages. Brush and floss often and begin cutting down on the bad habits that have led to a less than A-List Smile, such as eating too much sugar, smoking or drinking too much coffee or tea. Having a happy, healthy mouth before you commit to any one or more of these procedures will ensure that the process goes smoothly – and looks beautiful.

Dental Implants

No A-list celeb would be caught dead with visible missing teeth! Implants are the procedure of choice for replacing a tooth that has to be removed due to cavity, gum disease or traumatic injury. Patients with missing teeth are vulnerable to gum disease, loss of bone and potentially negative changes in facial structure. Dental implants provide an innovative way to minimize or eliminate these and other problems, while restoring function and beauty to patients' smiles.

Unlike traditional treatments for tooth loss, such as dentures and bridges, dental implants are actually fused to the jawbone, providing the most durable, long-lasting way to replace missing teeth. Implants are now considered to be "state-of the-art" and the "new standard of care" in dentistry for replacing missing teeth.

How does the procedure work?

Getting dental implants is a multi-step process beginning with the surgical placement of titanium posts into the jawbone under anesthesia. This procedure is usually performed by an oral surgeon or periodontist (gum specialist).

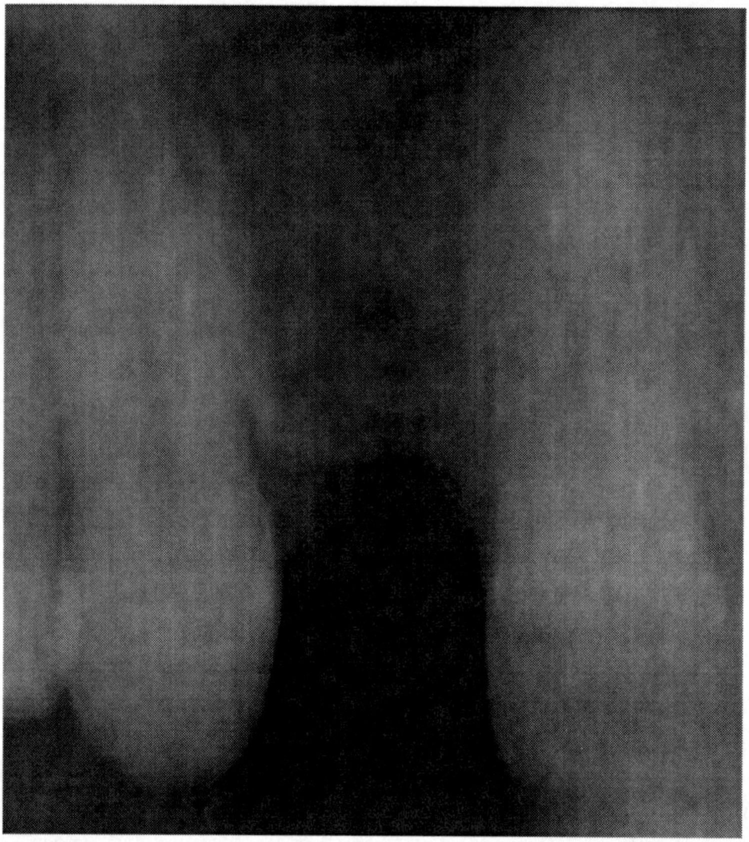

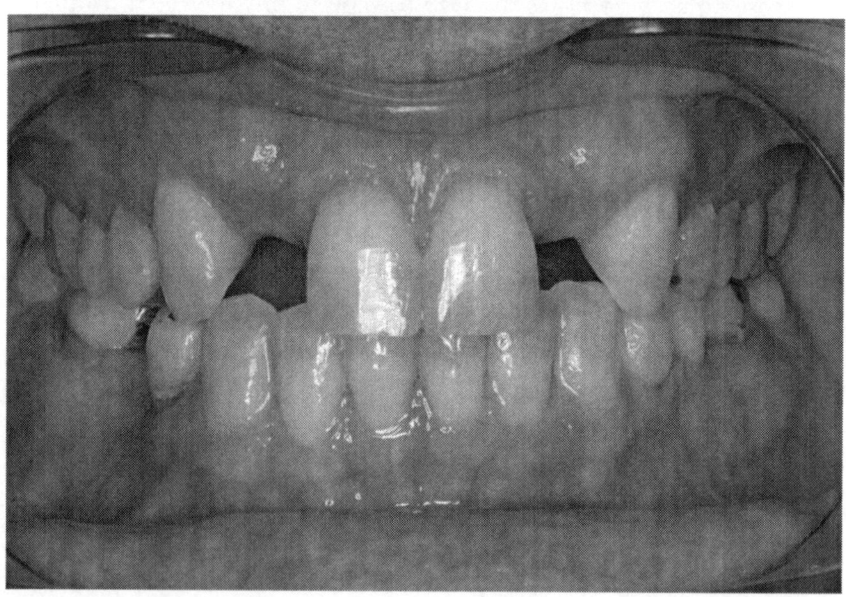

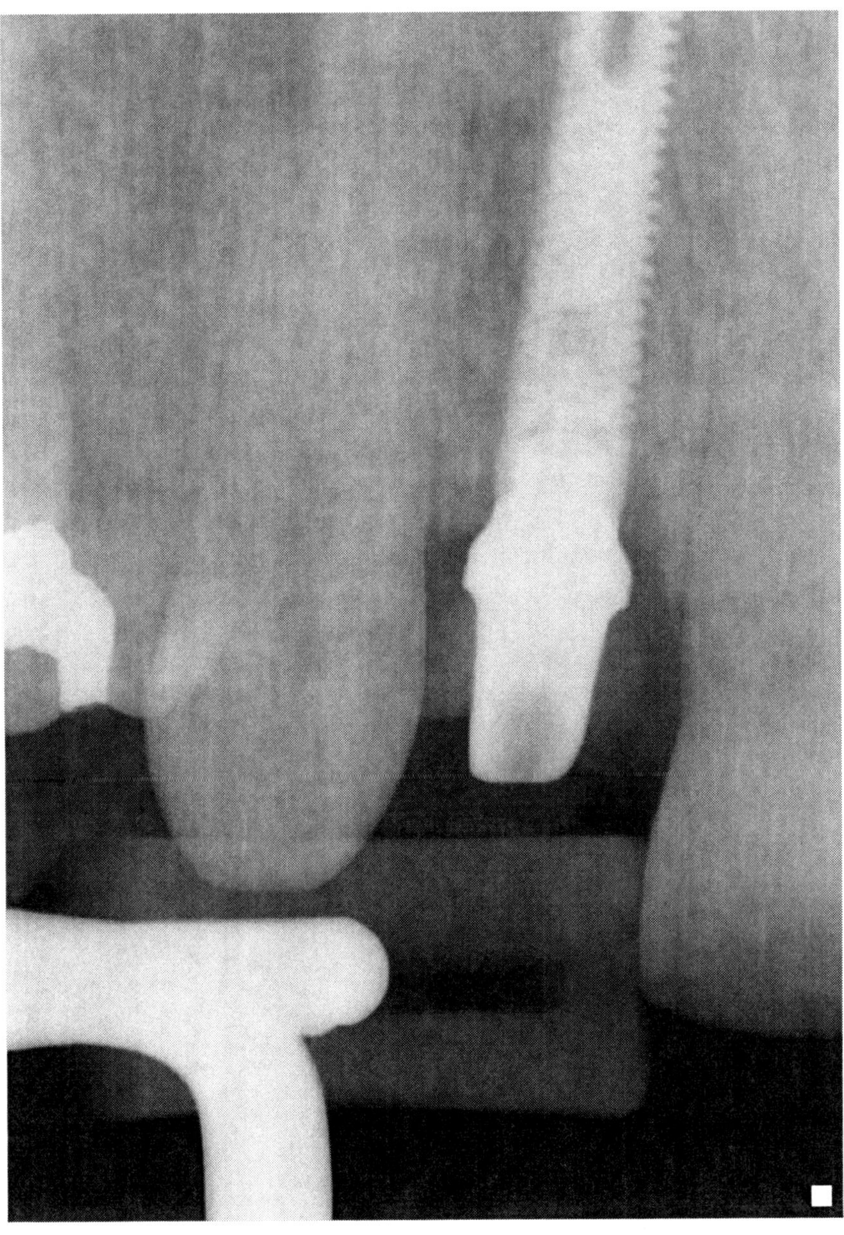

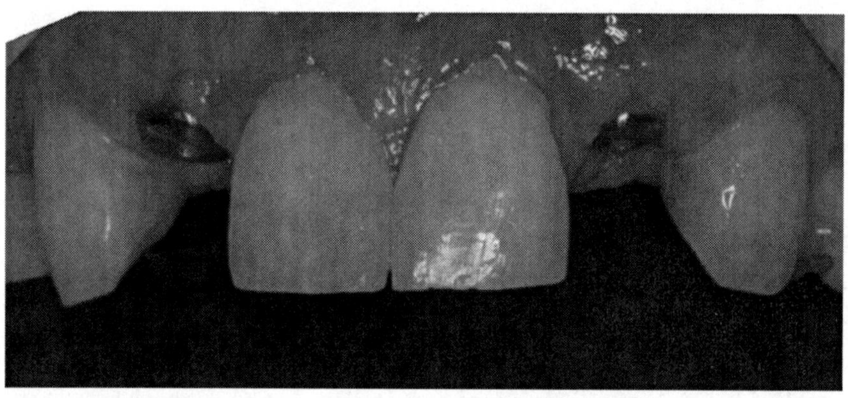

After several months of healing, these posts will have permanently fused to the jaw, enabling them to function like the roots of natural teeth. Next, your cosmetic dentist will make a putty molding of the implant and send it to the dental lab to order a custom made crown that attaches to the titanium posts.

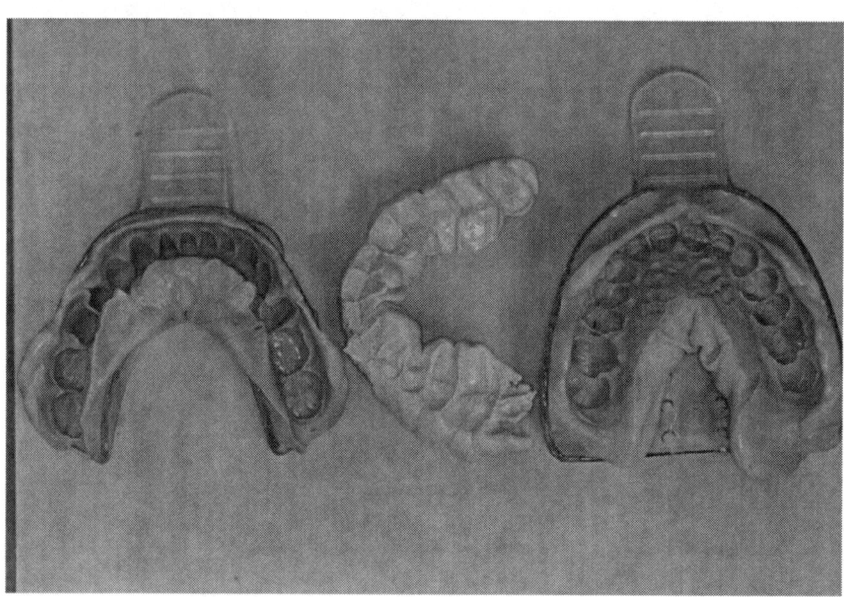

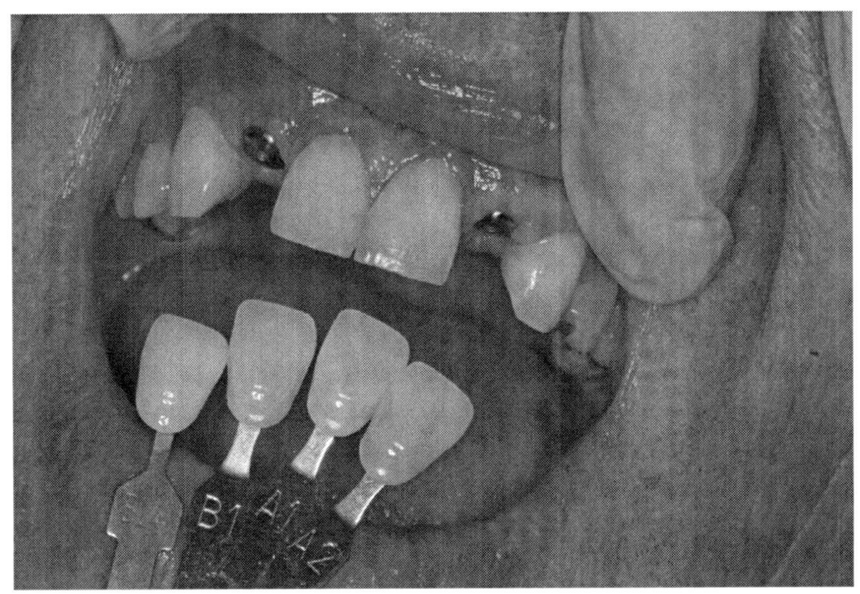
B1
A1
A2

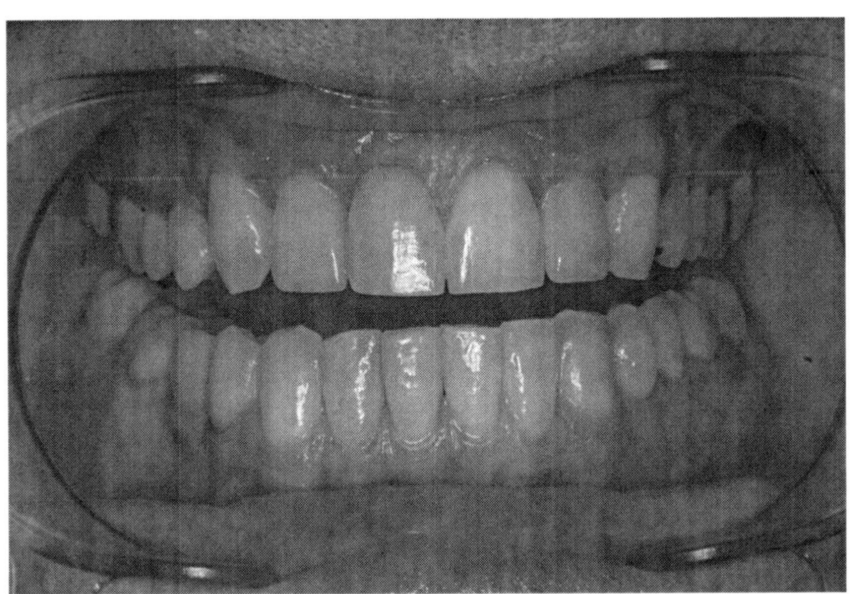

What are the pros and cons?

Every dental procedure comes with a list of pros and cons. Here are my thoughts concerning the pros and cons of dental implants:

- **Pros**: Unlike bridges and removable dentures, implants stand on their own and are not connected to or supported by surrounding teeth. Like your natural teeth, you can floss and clean normally around your implant. Specially designed to match the color and appearance of the rest of your smile, dental implants look, feel and function just like natural teeth. Also, replacing the tooth with an implant helps preserve the bone in the area of the extraction.
- **Cons**: Implants are the most costly option for replacing missing teeth. Because implants are surgically placed, the procedure is more invasive. If you are looking for a quick option for replacing your teeth for a special occasion, then implants are not your option. This procedure is more time-intensive than the alternative options of bridges and removable dentures.

How much will it cost?

Dental implants (including the crowns that screw into the implant) can vary in price depending on what region of the country you live. They can range from $2,000 up to $3,500 for each implant.

Will insurance cover this procedure?

Implants are generally not fully covered by dental insurance. The rules for each insurance plan may differ depending on the benefits package that you choose. Typically, insurance companies do not cover the implant surgery.

If your plan offers benefits for major services such as teeth replacements and crowns, they may cover your dental implants. If you want to be certain of the benefits offered by your plan before starting your work, your dentist may be willing to submit a letter with x-rays to your insurance to get a pre-authorization of the procedure with fees that they will pay as well as fees that will be due by you.

How long will it last?

Implants are permanent fixtures that can last a lifetime. Just like your natural teeth, implants must be cared for properly. Bacterial plaque and tarter can affect the bone surrounding the implant and cause it to loosen and fail. Daily brushing and flossing will help keep your implant stabilized. Your dental team can monitor the success of your implant during your routine dental visits for a professional cleaning and exam.

A-List Advice:

Don't stop with the pages of this book. Obviously, there is much more to learn than you can find here – or in any one resource – about all of these various dental products and procedures. So go to the library, visit dental websites and order brochures straight from the manufacturer in order to know everything you possibly can about every procedure you're interested in getting.

Bonding

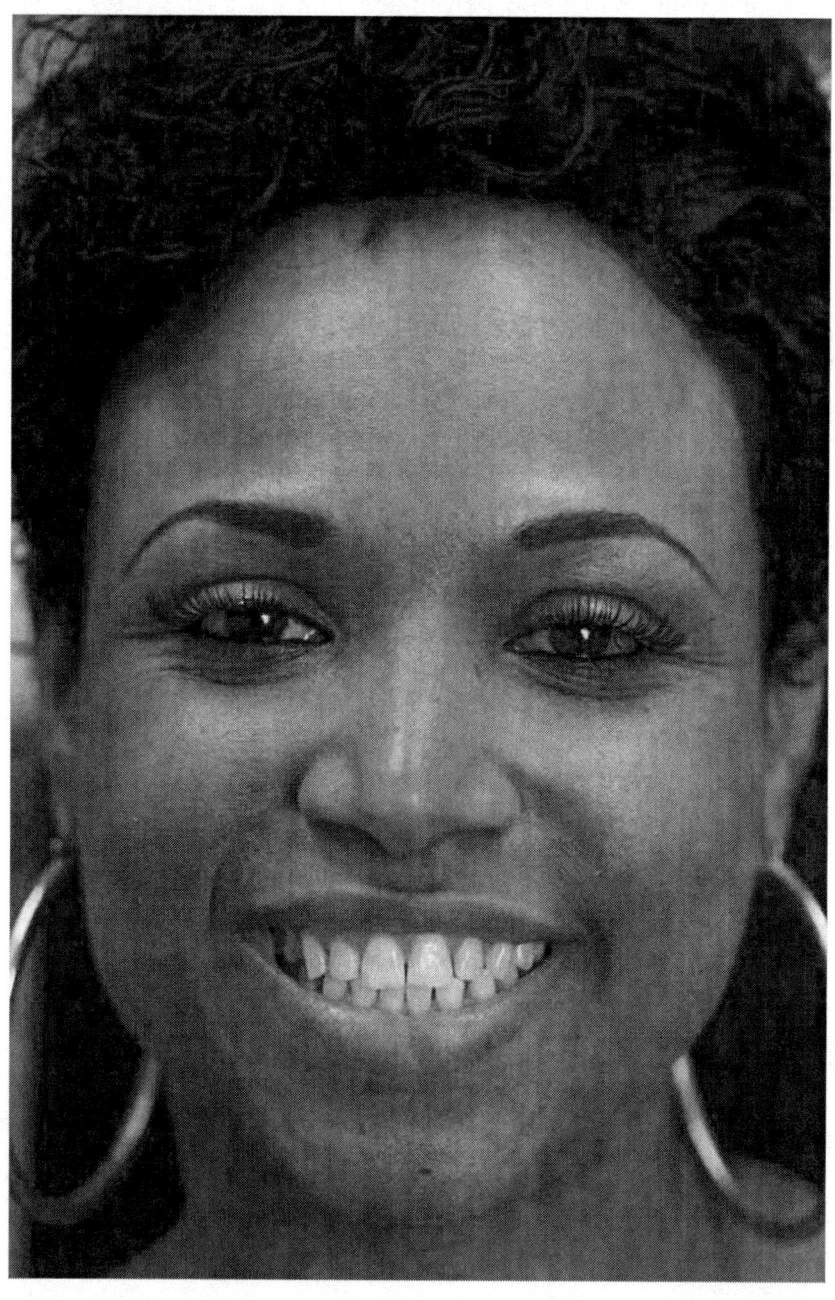

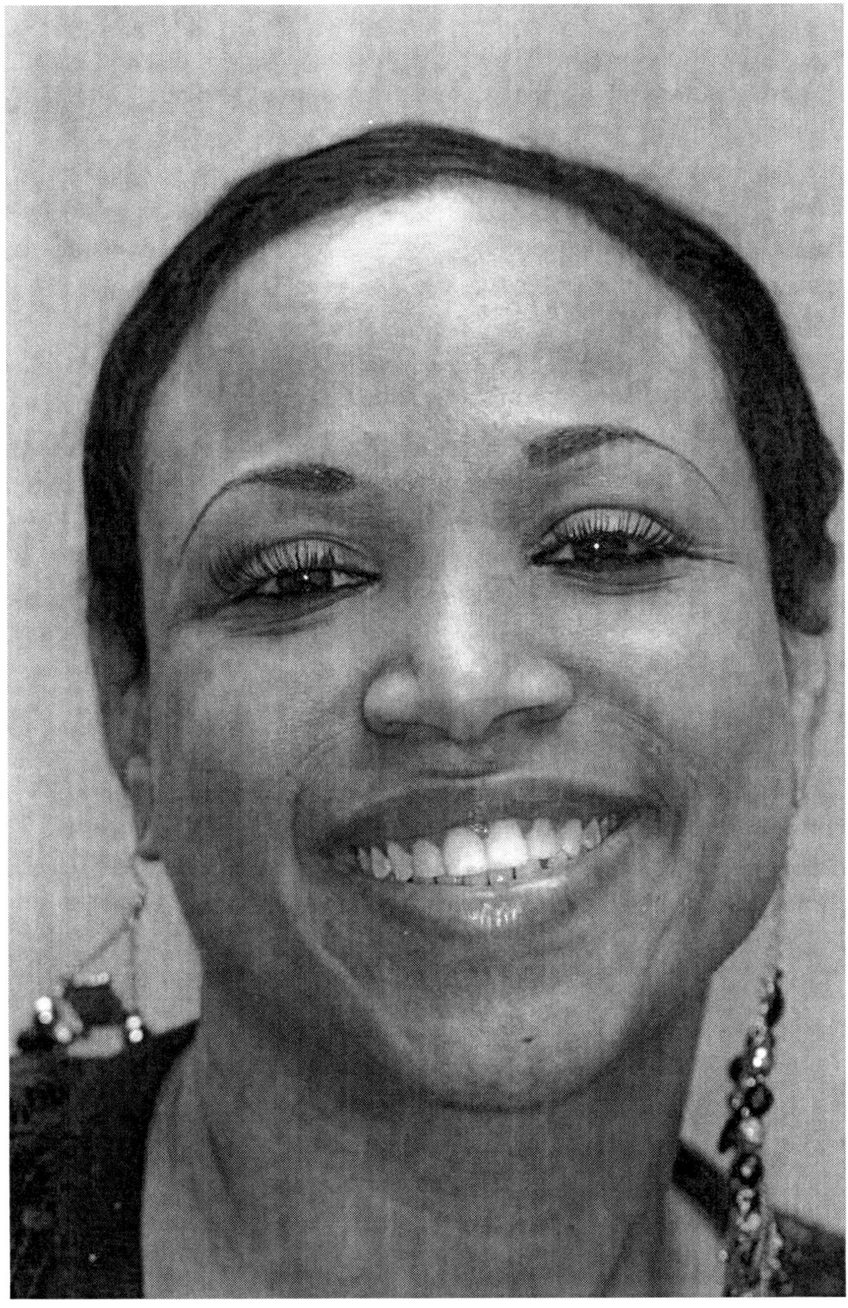

Another popular choice that A-list celebs turn to is bonding. Notables that have gotten bonding include hip-hop legend Nas. Dental bonding is used to address a variety of cosmetic and restorative dental issues.

Whether your teeth are chipped, cracked, discolored or decayed or you are concerned about small gaps between teeth or receding gums, dental bonding can provide a long-lasting solution to many of your dental problems. Dental bonding is typically the quickest, easiest and least expensive way to repair minor cosmetic imperfections in your smile.

How does the procedure work?

First, a mild acid is placed on the tooth to "open the pores" of the outer and inner tooth structure. Next, the dentist will place a liquid adhesive in the tooth that acts as a "glue" to hold the filling material inside the pores of the tooth. Your dentist will have the bonding material in his or her office and will select the color material that matches your tooth the best. The material comes in a variety of shades of white, yellow, grays, browns and translucents so that your dentist can create natural looking tooth.

Once the putty filling material is placed on the tooth, it is molded and shaped to achieve the desired result (i.e. repair the chip, close the space, lengthen the tooth, mask the localized discoloration, etc.). The filling is then secured and locked with an UV light, smoothed and polished to feel as normal as your original tooth felt.

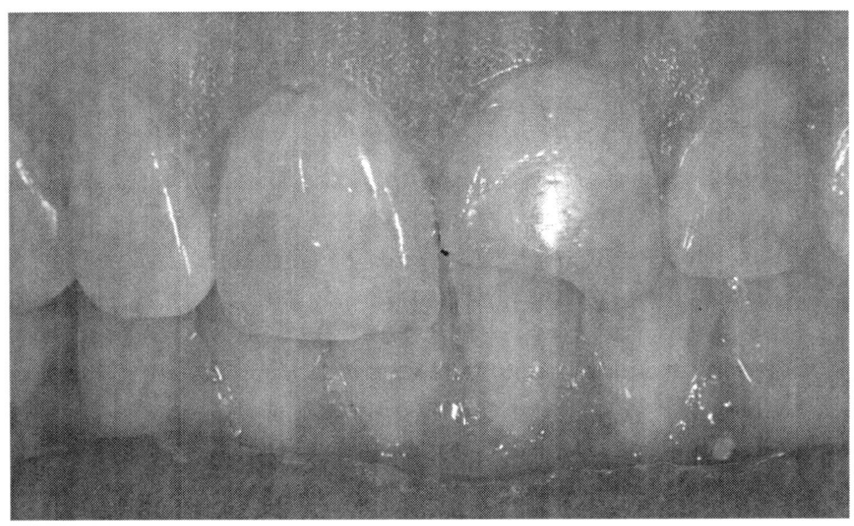

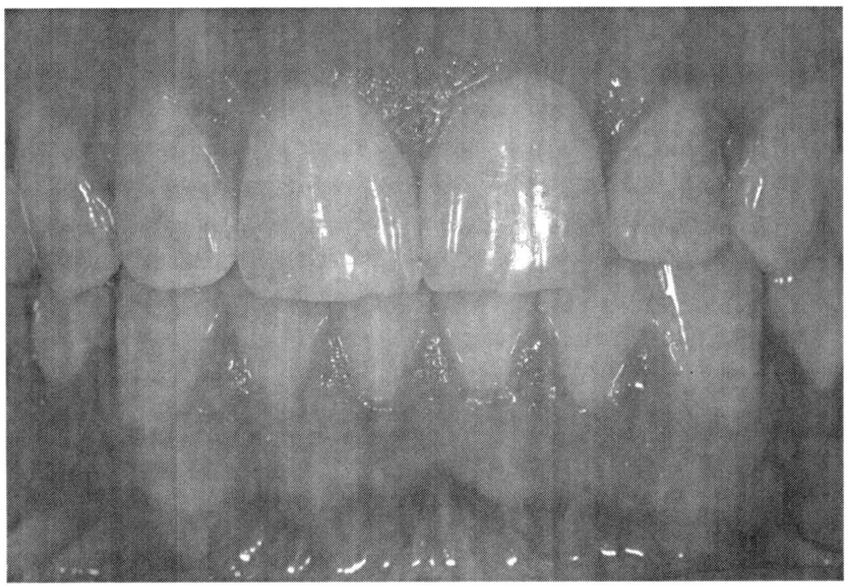

What are the pros and cons?

Every dental procedure comes with a list of pros and cons. Here are my thoughts concerning the pros and cons of dental bonding:

- **Pros**: Bonding is a conservative option to doing porcelain veneers. Unlike porcelain veneers, bonding is a procedure that does not always require extensive drilling and therefore the dentist can keep more of your healthy teeth structure. The fee for bonding is considerably less than porcelain veneers. Because your dentist has the bonding materials in-house, the procedure can be done in just one short visit.
- **Cons**: The results of dental bonding are dependant on how skilled your cosmetic dentist is. If your dentist is not highly artistic and doesn't have an eye for color, the results of your bonding may not look as natural and life-like as your natural tooth or porcelain veneers. The bonding material does not hold the luster of porcelain veneers and will, over time, begin to stain and discolor. As a result, the bonding may need to be replaced much sooner than desired. Although bonding materials are strong, they are not as strong as porcelain and may chip more easily.

How much will it cost?

You can expect to spend between $250 and $500, per tooth, for dental bonding.

Will insurance cover this procedure?

Dental bondings placed on the front teeth are generally partially covered by dental insurance. The rules for each insurance plan may differ depending on the benefits package that you choose. If your plan offers benefits for services such as plastic composite resin fillings, then they may cover your bondings. If you want to be certain of the benefits offered by your plan before starting your work, your dentist may be willing to submit a letter with x-rays to your insurance to get a pre-authorization of the procedure with fees that they will pay as well as fees that will be covered by you.

How long will it last?

The average life span of bondings are 3-5 years but can last up to a decade with proper care.

> **A-List Advice:**
>
> *Take notes! It's okay; there are a lot of procedures in this section and I want you to keep track of them all. If you don't have a notebook handy, scribble in the margins. It's okay, this is one book I WANT you to write, doodle and draw in! After all, your A-List Smile depends on it.*

Put Your Money Where Your Mouth Is:

How to Pay for Your A-List Smile

I, for one, believe that price should never be an issue when pursuing an A-List Smile. Your looks, your health and your emotional well-being are too important to give up on your dreams because of a few dollars and sense – even a lot of dollars and sense. This section will help reassure you that there will always be a way to pay for your A-List Smile, even if it takes a little paperwork, patience and practicality.

Smile Now – Pay Later!

Throughout this chapter we talked extensively about what procedures may or may not be covered by insurance. Most cosmetic or A-List procedures are *not* covered – or at least, covered fully – by insurance. The most popular option that people are turning to in order finance their dental procedures is called CareCredit®.

Why do doctors offer CareCredit? According to the company website, "Many patients put off treatments and procedures because they cannot afford to pay. Doctors offer CareCredit payment plans as a convenient option to normal credit cards, cash or checks. CareCredit allows the patient to pay over time often without incurring interest charges instead of a lump sum prior to treatment. Removing the cost barrier often allows clinicians to focus on optimal treatment for the patient. Not all doctors offer every CareCredit plan. Once you are a

CareCredit cardholder you can discuss with your doctor which plan works best for you and your budget."

Endorsed by the American Dental Association, the Society for Excellence in Eyecare and the American Society of Plastic Surgeons, CareCredit is offered in dental offices throughout the country. It offers up to 18 months of no-interest financing and then 11.90% financing up to 5 years. CareCredit can also be used for medical expenses, eyeglasses and in veterinary offices as well. For more information, visit www.carecredit.com.

According to their website, "You can apply online or download and print the application and take it to your healthcare provider. The application is quick and easy, and after it's submitted, you'll instantly learn if you're approved. CareCredit is accepted by over 100,000 providers and is the nation's leading financing program... You can search by your doctor's name, or if you don't have a doctor in mind, you can search for doctors in your area by using the ZIP code search option."

Other dental financing companies include Capital One and Chase. The above options will allow you to "smile now and pay for it later"! What next? From dental schools to government programs, if the timing is right and you fit certain criteria, you may be able to qualify for a variety of the programs listed below. The information that follows is courtesy of The National Institute of Dental and Craniofacial Research (NIDCR), one of the federal government's National Institutes of Health:

Dental Schools (Take One)

Dental schools can be a good source of quality, reduced-cost dental treatment. Most of these teaching facilities have clinics that allow dental students to gain experience treating patients while providing care at a reduced cost. Experienced, licensed dentists closely supervise the students. Post-graduate and faculty clinics are also available at most schools. [**Source**: *NIH Publication No. 07-6097*] (In my Resources section, I have a full list of dental schools across the country, arranged by state.)

Bureau of Primary Health Care

The Bureau of Primary Health Care, a service of the Health Resources and Services Administration (HRSA), supports federally-funded community health centers across the country that provide free or reduced-cost health services, including dental care. To obtain a list of centers in your area, contact the HRSA Information Center toll-free at 1-888-ASK-HRSA (1-888-275-4772) or visit their web site at http://ask.hrsa.gov/pc/. [**Source**: *NIH Publication No. 07-6097*]

One note: when getting discounted dental care at either dental schools or training programs, make sure to check with your insurance carrier first to determine how much, if any, is covered. For instance, while dental schools may provide cosmetic dentistry, Primary Care may not cover it unless it's corrective.

State and Local Resources

Your state or local health department may know of programs in your area that offer free or reduced-cost dental care. Call your local or state health department to learn more about their financial assistance programs. Check your local telephone book for the number to call. [**Source**: *NIH Publication No. 07-6097*]

When All Else Fails: *Dr. Austin's Top-7 Favorite Tips for Free, Reduced or Affordable Dental Care*

Where can one start if you really don't have any money to pay for the products and procedures listed here? I know scouring the web, hitting the pavement and filling out paperwork to pay for your dental procedures can be exhausting, frustrating work.

Most frustrating of all is that you may make too much to qualify for this program but not enough to qualify for another; when trying to gain funding – or even access to funding – for dental care there can be as many ways to keep you from resources as there are resources themselves.

So before you give up completely, check out my following seven favorite tips for getting the funding you need for the A-List Smile you deserve:

1.) Get creative: Most dental offices take major credit cards. BUT... most will even give a standard discount of 5% (or more) if you pay in full with cash or check before you start the procedure. If it's too much for your pocketbook to get all the procedures at once, spread the necessary work over time. If that doesn't work, go discount: Costco bulk discount stores offer dental care in some locations.

2.) Seek charity: Here are a few dental charities/programs that offer qualified candidates free dental care:

- Smiles For Success (American Association of Women Dentists)
- Give Back A Smile (American Academy of Cosmetic Dentists)

3.) Find training: Thanks to the National Institute of Dental and Craniofacial Research, you already know that dental schools offer reduced fees for dental services, but did you know that certain training hospitals in each state will have dental residency programs where readers can also get reduced fees for dental services? Services are provided by dentists who have graduated and are licensed (in most cases).

4.) **Negotiate wisely**: When all else fails, it doesn't hurt to negotiate or barter with your dentist if you have a service or skill to offer! For instance, maybe you are a carpenter and your dentist needs office repairs.

5.) **"Plan" ahead**: If your company doesn't offer a dental plan, ask them to join a plan but tell them you and your co-workers will pay 100% of the premium. You'll save by getting a group rate and have an easier time than looking for an individual plan.

6.) **When All Else (Really) Fails** – *Clinical Trials*: NIDCR sometimes seeks volunteers with specific dental, oral and craniofacial conditions to participate in research studies, also known as clinical trials. Researchers may provide study participants with limited free or low-cost dental treatment for the particular condition they are studying. To find out if there are any NIDCR clinical trials that you might fit into, visit the NIDCR web site at http://www.nidcr.nih.gov/ and click on "NIDCR Studies Seeking Patients." For a complete list of all federally funded clinical trials, visit http://clinicaltrials.gov. If you do not have access to the Internet, you may need to visit your local library or ask a friend or family member for assistance. To see if you qualify for any clinical trials being conducted at the Bethesda, Maryland, campus, you can call the Clinical Center's Patient Recruitment and Public Liaison Office at 1-800-411-1222. [**Source:** *NIH Publication No. 07-6097*]

7.) **Lay-away or pre-pay for your smile:** When it comes to getting an A-List Smile, timing really IS everything. If you can plan – and budget – ahead, it might be a good idea for you to lay-away – in other words, pre-pay – for your dental procedures. That's right; you can actually prepay for your smile by sending in payments in advance of starting the treatment. Once you've sent the dentist the agreed amount, they can begin the work.

> *"A beautiful smile leaves such a lasting impression!"*
>
> ~ **Mary Mary**

Step 5:

Care For Your A-List Smile

"Wrinkles should merely indicate where smiles have been."

~ Mark Twain

Getting an A-List Smile is only half the battle; caring for your A-List Smile assures that the confidence you feel now won't wane or lapse as a result of insufficient or negligent care once the excitement dies down and routine sets in. I recognize that dentistry is not the most popular of procedures for my patients. I also know that "out of sight, out of mind" definitely applies when it comes to recent dental procedures.

Patients often think that one procedure is enough, or that once a procedure is done, that's it; there's no need for proper care and maintenance. But as fitness trainers tell their clients all the time, "You didn't gain all this weight overnight; you're not going to lose it overnight, either." In other words, maintaining an A-List Smile is a full-time job. Here are a few ways *5 Steps to a Hollywood A-List Smile* can help:

- **Proper Cleaning Procedures**
- **Healthy Cleaning Habits on the Go**

- **Proper Care and Maintenance for the A-List Smile:** *Product by Product*
- **What next?**

In many ways, this is one of the book's most important chapters. After all, what good is an A-List Smile if you don't care for it? The best part about this chapter is that, unlike getting an A-List Smile, caring for one doesn't have to time-intensive, painful or even expensive.

The main thing to remember when preparing to care for your new smile is to create good, solid habits built around a daily routine of sensible and timely intervention techniques that both foster healthy oral care plus the specific requirements dictated by your new smile.

Many of my patients think that just because they've got a new A-List Smile their work is done; nothing could be further from the truth. In fact, now is where the real work begins. Remember that lack of interest and bad habits may have helped contribute to your less-than A-List Smile in the first place; don't repeat history just because your dental work is now done.

Much like the confidence gained from having a great smile is built on good habits and positive emotions, so too is caring for your A-List Smile. Dental care is a process that comes from forming good habits.

Human nature is hard to change; we are creatures of habit – both good and bad habits! If you didn't care for your smile before, you won't do it now just because you have a prettier smile. If you do it at all, it will be because you've made up your mind to change what you're doing for yourself in every way.

View this not just as an opportunity to close the door on good oral healthcare but to throw it wide open and really take advantage of your new smile by building healthy, hopeful habits to keep it A-List for the rest of your life.

A-List Advice:

Health = habits! I want you to remember this equation as you read forward and uncover the secrets to caring for an A-List Smile. The better your smile habits are, the cleaner your mouth will be and the healthier YOU will be.

Proper Cleaning Procedures

Just because you now have an A-List Smile don't think that you can ignore the basics: brushing, flossing and proper nutrition are the backbone of any healthy smile, and shouldn't be ignored just because you've been to the dentist four times in the last two months to polish off your A-List Smile:

Brush-a-Brush

Regardless of whether you have Invisalign, a Snap-On Smile, dental bonding, implants, porcelain veneers or other procedures that may improve your smile, brushing your teeth will become an integral part of keeping an A-List Smile for as long as possible.

While certain appliances such as Invisalign clear braces or Snap-On Smiles might require special, extra cleaning procedures (see the next section for specific notes on proper care and procedures), don't forget the basics: brush twice a day with a soft or an electric toothbrush, and be persistent about it.

The proper brushing technique is to hold your brush at a 45-degree angle toward the gum line. The goal is to remove cavity causing and gum disease causing plaque that may be hiding below the gums. Make sure to brush the front, biting and tongue surfaces of your teeth. Total brushing time per brushing session should be two minutes.

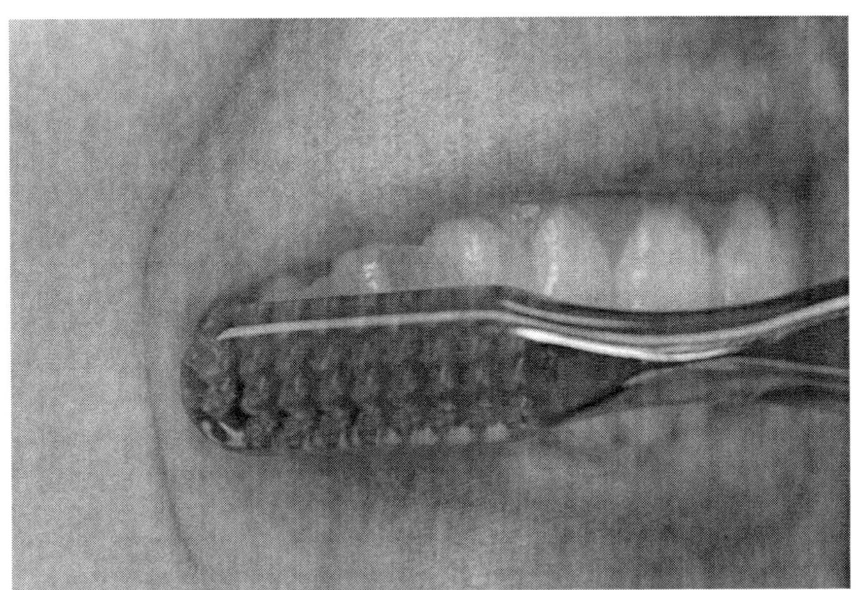

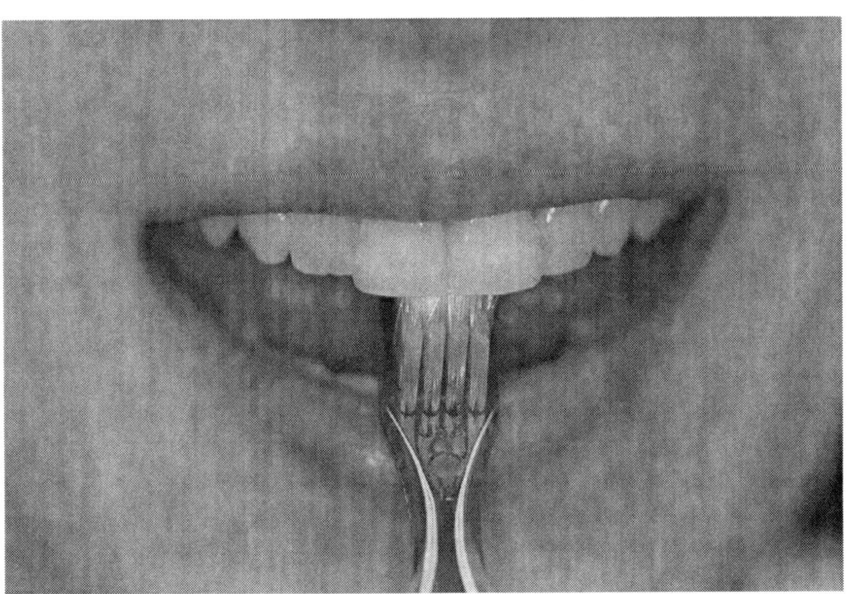

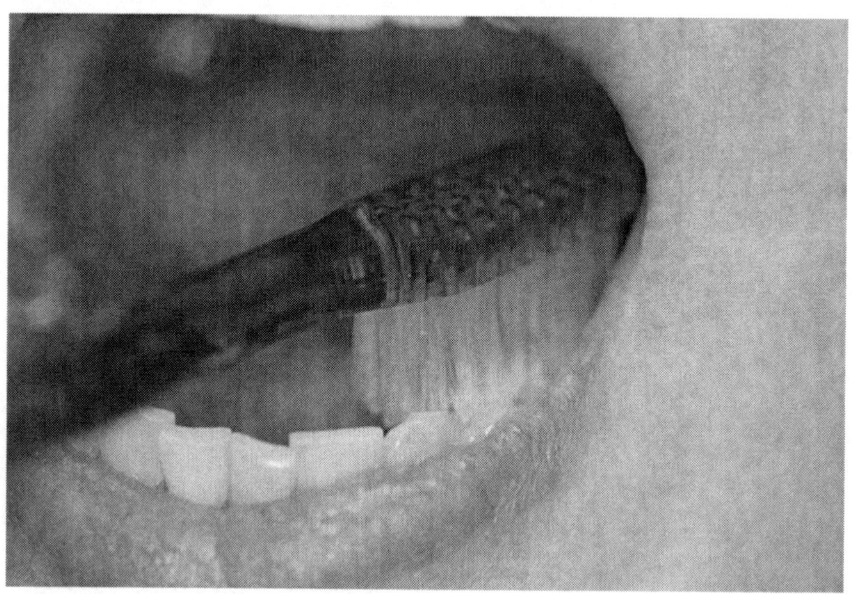

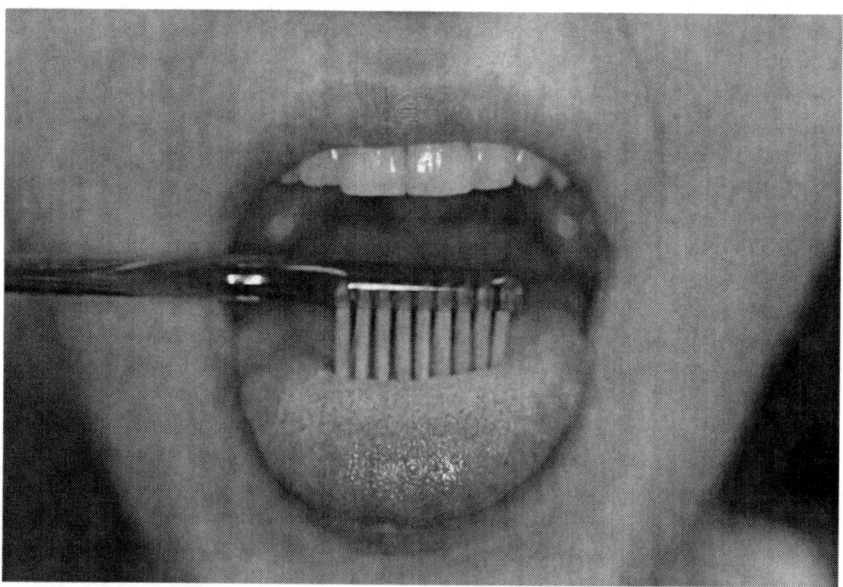

Getting an A-List Smile should motivate you to care for your teeth even more than before, and if you feel your resolve lagging try this simple trick: look in the mirror! The best way to stay motivated about keeping an A-List Smile is to see it, front and center, every day.

Floss Away

Flossing your teeth regularly, at least once a day, is a vital tool for saving your new A-List Smile. Flossing will help clean the surfaces between your teeth and below the gums where your toothbrush reaches. It is THE SECRET WEAPON to preventing cavities from forming between your natural teeth or under your veneers or bonding. Flossing also reaches areas below the gums to prevent gum disease from developing, which leads to tooth loss.

The proper flossing technique is to hold the floss around your fingers, gently place the floss between your teeth, hold the floss against the tooth to form a "C" around the tooth. Then gently move the floss "up and down" in a vertical motion. Just a few seconds between each tooth will help you save your smile.

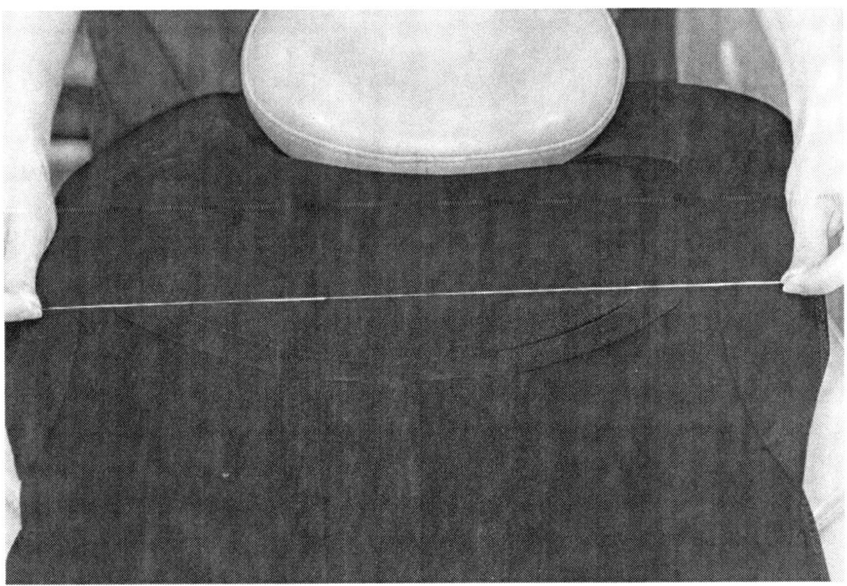

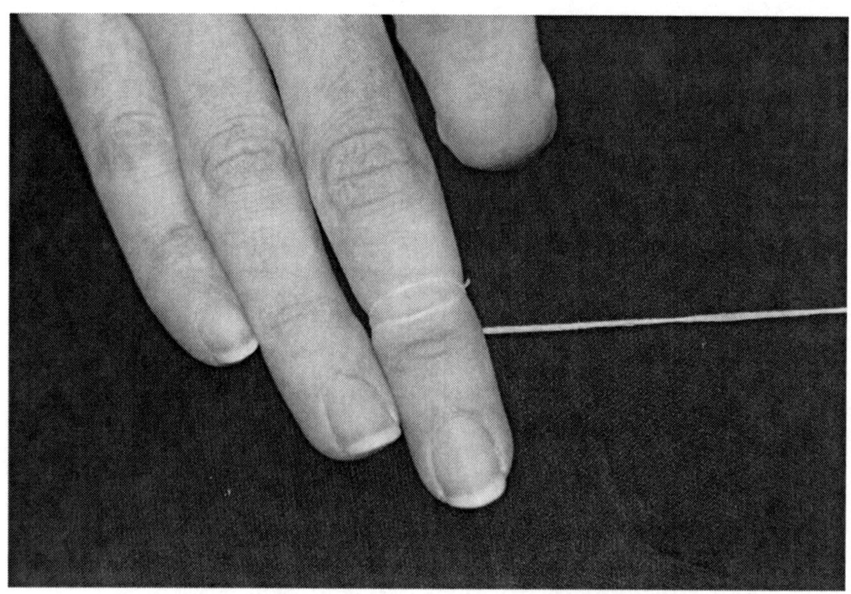

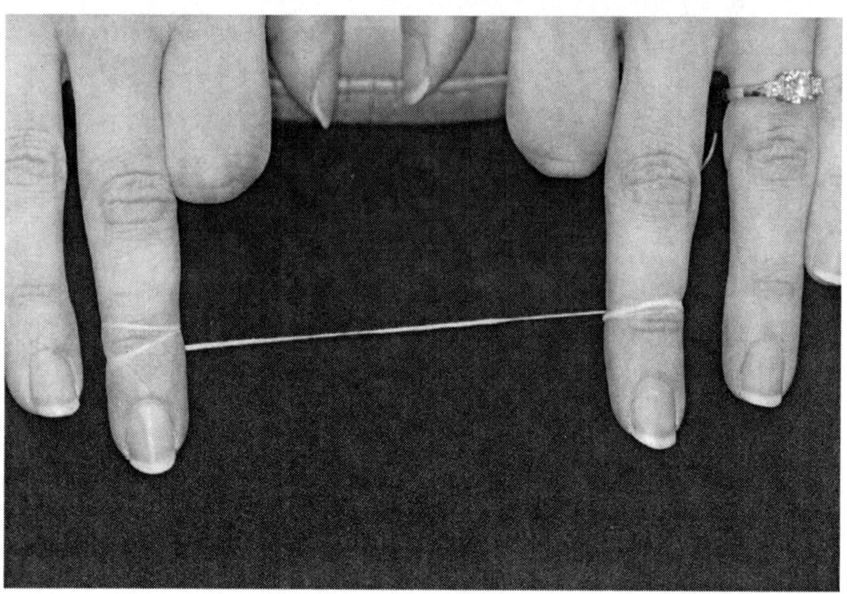

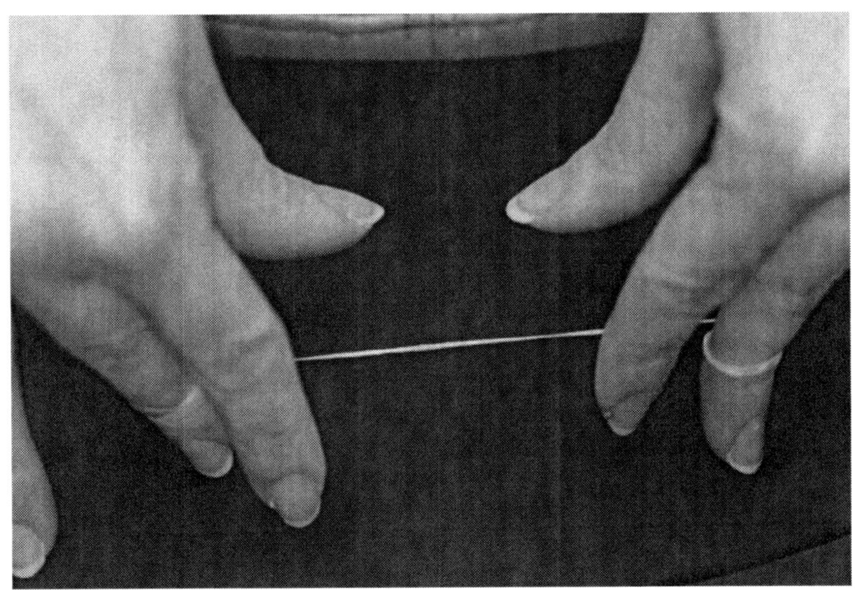

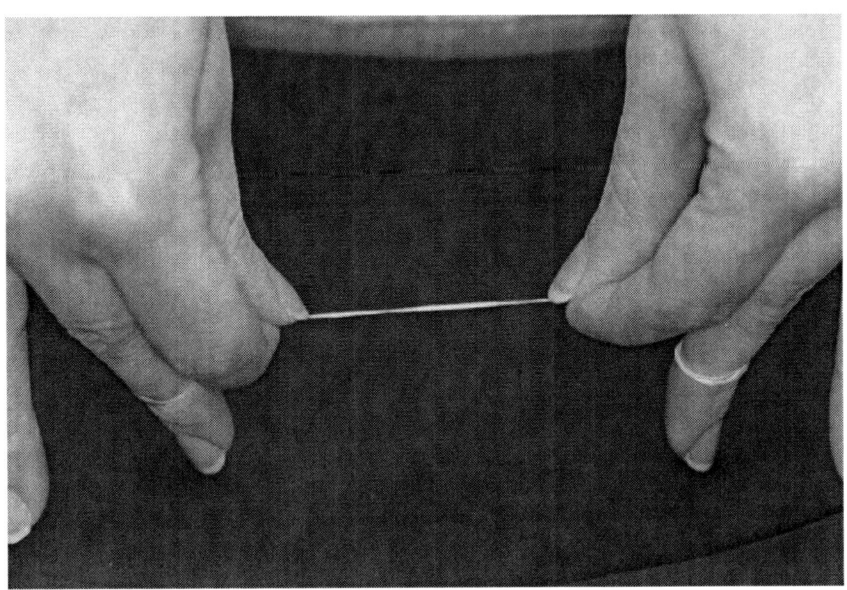

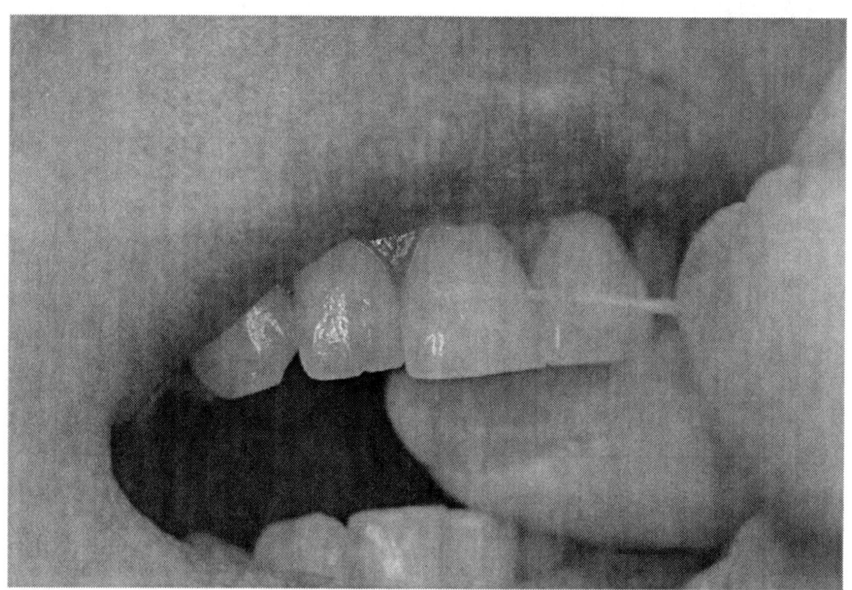

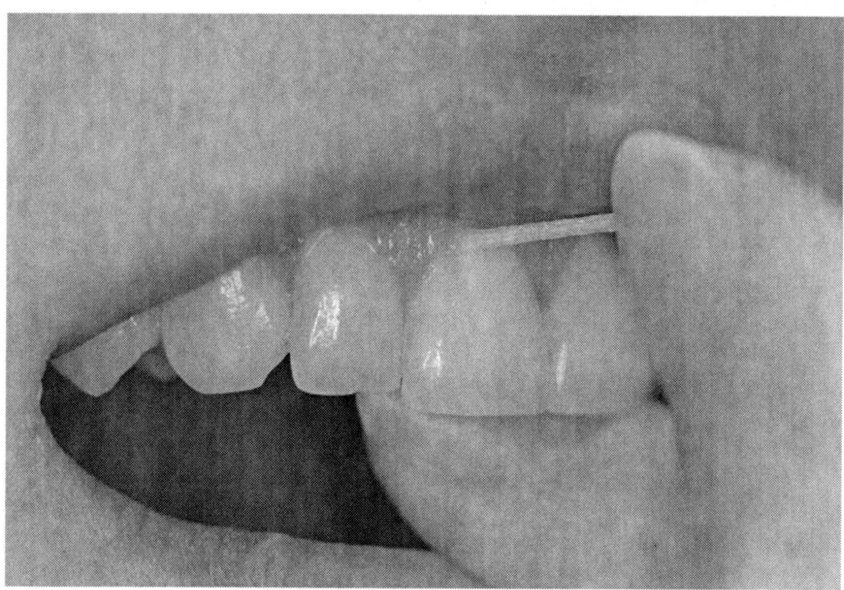

Many people choose to skip this important step of flossing because it seems like an extra step and time consuming. Others find that the whole process of holding and manipulating the floss is difficult and cumbersome. My favorite find has been those great pre-loaded floss handles that are sold by the bags. They are so easy to use. Instead of wrapping the floss around your fingers, just simply hold the handle against the tooth to form a "C" around the tooth. Then gently move the floss "up and down" in a vertical motion. Again, just a few seconds between each tooth is all you need.

Don't Forget Nutrition

Many patients think that if they merely brush and floss they can eat whatever they want, but nothing could be further from the truth. I like to school them on the "holy tooth trinity," or:

1. **Brushing**
2. **Flossing**
3. **Dining**

By eating right, you can increase the health and longevity of an A-List Smile long past its warranty date. By eating poorly, your new A-List Smile could go straight-to-video in no time, literally undoing all the hard work, effort, time and money you spent in obtaining an A-List Smile in the first place.

Test Your Knowledge on Foods That Can Ruin an A-List Smile

Keeping an A-List Smile can be simple if you make the right food choices. Let's test your knowledge on foods that can ruin your smile.

✓ Check the option below that can put your smile on the D-list:

_____ **Processed cereals: cereals like Frosted Flakes and Fruit Loops as well as "plain" cereals such as Wheaties, Cheerios, etc.**

_____ **Cake**

_____ **Candy**

_____ Chocolate drinks, chocolate milk, cocoa

_____ Condensed milk

_____ Cookies

_____ Canned fruit (with syrup)

_____ Dried fruit (including raisins)

_____ Graham crackers

_____ Gum

_____ Ice cream

_____ Fruit juices (that aren't 100% juice)

_____ Imitation fruit juices (including Hi-C)

_____ Jelly, jam

_____ Macaroni

_____ Marshmallows

_____ Pastries

_____ Pie

_____ Soda

_____ Sweet toppings, sauces, syrups, icings

_____ White bread (including hot dog and hamburger buns)

_____ Caramel corn

_____ Crackers such as Ritz, Bacon Thins, Twigs, etc.

_____ Doughnuts

_____ Honey

_____ Jell-O and gelatin

_____ **Kool-Aid**

_____ **Malted milk**

_____ **Milk shakes**

_____ **Molasses**

_____ **Peanut butter (Jif, Skippy, et al.)**

_____ **Processed cheeses**

_____ **Puddings**

_____ **Tang**

_____ **Waffles, pancakes**

How do you think you did? If you checked all of the above and only consume these foods and beverages in moderation, then you're on the road to keeping a healthy, A-List Smile.

Many foods and beverages that may seem harmless often times are high in sugar or carbohydrates that quickly convert to cavity forming acids in the mouth. Get in the habit of reading nutritional labels to help you make the best choices to help you have an "A-List" smile.

In general, avoid the usual suspects like candy, sugar, sodas and other sweet treats. A rare indulgence now and then shouldn't send you running into the arms of your dental professional, but bad habits lead to bad teeth, so keep those indulgences to a bare minimum.

In addition to these basic guidelines, here are a few specific suggestions on how proper nutrition can benefit your new A-List Smile:

- **Avoid starchy or "sticky" foods**: You know what the bacteria on your teeth and tongue and in your mouth feed on? Carbohydrates. So the fewer carbs you eat, the less "food" your bacteria get to thrive on. By no means am I telling you to limit or restrict carbohydrates from your daily diet; they are a vital tool for providing your body with the energy and resources it needs daily. However, eating carbohydrates to excess – starchy, "sticky" foods like bread, cakes, cookies, brownies and pies – can put your mouth at risk.

- **Eat first, drink second**: We are a nation that thrives on convenience, but did you know that fruit juice is mostly sugar? In fact, it takes eight whole apples to equal the sugar content in one glass of apple juice. So while drinking juice may be convenient, eating a piece of fruit rather than drinking a glass of fruit juice can not only reduce the amount of sugar you ingest – which as we all know is bad for your teeth – but can help make you feel fuller at the same time.
- **Get your vitamins**: Your teeth can decay when there are not enough vitamins, nutrients and minerals consumed for proper dental care. Eating properly doesn't just help keep your mouth clean and free of bacteria; it also helps make your teeth stronger. For instance, Vitamin-C can contribute to stronger, healthier teeth, as can calcium. So make sure you eat properly and take a quality vitamin supplement to ensure you're getting enough of what your body needs every single day.

Routines to Last a Lifetime

What you do is important; how you do things is equally important. For instance, brushing your teeth twice a day and flossing once a day is great – but not if you can only get motivated enough to do so on Monday or Tuesday before giving up for the rest of the week.

Many of my patients leave my office often vowing to brush twice and floss once every day; and they do so, for a week or two. Then old habits die hard, and they settle into the familiar routine of brushing once or twice a day and flossing once or twice – before their next dental visit!

Relax; I am not here to scold you, lecture you or nag you about brushing and flossing regularly. I know other dentists have probably been there and done that. However, I am here to give you the good news: good habits are as easy to practice as bad ones and, even better, they last forever!

If you're having a hard time fitting proper dental care into your routine, you're not alone; many of my patients find it just as difficult to care for their teeth properly. That's why I've come up with the following quick tips to help you replace bad habits with good ones, and care for your new A-List Smile every day:

- **Out with the old, in with the new**: You need to identify your bad habits before you can replace them. So take some time now to pinpoint your top five or, if you have that many, your top ten worst habits. They can range from not brushing your teeth at night to using mouthwash instead of brushing to eating too much candy and/or soda and so on. But the sooner you recognize what bad habits you're dealing with, the sooner you'll know what you have to do to replace them with good ones.
- **Replace for your face**: Healthy eating isn't always easy. Convenient, junk, fast and just plain bad food is easier to get, prepare, buy and eat than food that's good for you. I understand that. So instead of trying to cut out every bad food, instead replace just one bad food a meal with something healthier. For instance, if you eat two donuts for breakfast every day, why not try replacing one of those donuts with an apple tomorrow? It may not entirely undo the damage you cause with the one donut you're still eating, but the healthy apple can go a long way toward rectifying the damage two donuts might have done. Chances are, as you practice this habit, you will eventually do away with donuts altogether.
- **Timing is everything**: If brushing and flossing regularly is conflicting with your schedule, take a look at WHY there is a conflict in the first place and what you can do about it. For instance, maybe you were taught as a child – as so many of us were – to brush your teeth just before bed. Well, if you're too tired at bedtime to brush and floss, don't wait so long; reverse the trend and brush and floss right after you eat dinner. This is just one of many ways where simply changing a habit or mindset can literally help you form a new habit – for life.
- **Publish your progress**: Remember how when you were a kid your parents used to proudly place your artwork, spelling test or good grade of the day on the fridge? Well, don't be afraid to

do the same for your good habits. Make a chart and keep track of your progress, even adding a gold star for every day you brush twice and floss once. Sure, it may seem hokey at first but give yourself a month and chances are, your little chart might just turn into one great, big habit!

A-List Advice:

They say "practice makes perfect," but actually only "perfect practice makes perfect." This means that if you practice something wrong – like using the wrong type of brush for your A-List Smile— you can actually do more harm than good. So by all means practice, but remember to practice perfect for optimum results.

Healthy Cleaning Habits on the Go

Let's face it: we're a country on the go. We travel for business and pleasure. We travel at night, on weekends and over holidays. We travel to celebrate, to explore, to educate and to edify. And whether our jaunts take a weekend, a week, a day or a month, we often leave one thing behind as we're packing our bags and boarding our flight: the proper, healthy cleaning habits we practice at home.

It's as if the minute we hit the road, we forget all we've learned about dental health and cleaning. Part of this is simply the busy nature of our travel activities. I mean, after a long day at a conference, business meeting or client presentation, the last thing you want to do is brush your teeth, let alone floss. And after a late night out exploring the sights, sounds, tastes and experiences of a foreign country, exhaustion often gets the upper hand over dentition.

In this section I share with you the secrets to making on the go smile care as simple as (steps) one, two and three:

Step # 1:

Travel Size It

If "not enough room in your luggage" is your standard excuse for not cleaning your teeth on the go, then you're in for some bad news: nowadays there are travel sizes of everything, from deodorant to mouthwash. So here are some quick fixes for you:

- **Bring travel sizes of toothpaste, mouthwash, dental floss and your toothbrush**
- **Bring your own toothbrush and floss and share toothpaste with your traveling partner**
- **Designate a zippered pocket or pouch in your luggage and ALWAYS keep it stocked with dental healthcare products; this will make it harder for you to forget each time you travel**

Step # 2:

Store and Go

On the go doesn't always mean frequent flyer miles and first-class tickets. Sometimes merely burning the midnight oil at work or working weekends can keep us from healthy brushing, flossing and even eating habits.

It's late, you're tired and where are you going to find a toothbrush at work, let alone dental floss? You're hungry, it's dark and it's easier to eat something quick, starchy and "sticky" out of the vending machine downstairs than tread out into the world for a healthier, heartier meal.

Well, here are some quick tips to help you take care of your new A-List Smile even while you're taking care of business:

- **Have an extra toothbrush, tube of toothpaste, roll of dental floss and bottle of mouthwash at/in your desk/office**
- **Schedule time to care for your teeth if you know you're going to be working late**
- **Pre-prepare healthy snacks like fresh fruit, cheese or nuts for those times when the vending machine is calling**

Step # 3:

Your Own Personal On-the-Go Kit

No matter where you go, how far you travel or how long you work, caring for an A-List Smile doesn't have to play second fiddle to the Eiffel Tower or that new marketing campaign you have to prepare by tomorrow morning. All you need is a little preparation, some forethought, some extras and you've got your very own on-the-go solution for your busy, on-the-go lifestyle.

Your Personal On-the-Go Kit should contain the following items:

- **A carrying case, plastic bag or re-sealable Tupperware style container (for storing items)**
- **Travel toothbrush (and sanitary lid)**
- **Tube of toothpaste**
- **Dental floss**
- **Mouthwash**
- **Hand sanitizer (before using dental floss)**
- **Handy wipes or extra napkins for easy clean-up**

A-List Advice:

Always be prepared to care for your A-List Smile on the go. Nowadays they have dental care products in every shape and size, including travel-size dental floss, mouthwash and even toothbrushes. Just the other day I saw a one-use toothbrush, complete with toothpaste already in the bristles, for sale at the gas station! Nowadays, there is simply NO excuse for not caring for your smile on the road.

Proper Care and Maintenance for the A-List Smile:

Procedure by Procedure

How to care for which procedure, how often and how thoroughly? Relax; I've got you covered. In this section I review the various A-List procedures that I discussed in the last section and share with you any special considerations there may be for your specific needs:

- **Porcelain Veneers:** Veneers can be brushed, and flossed, just like your regular teeth. So the same healthy routines you had before – brushing, flossing and regular dental visits – still apply. The only special recommendation I would make is to invest in a night guard to avoid any unnecessary grinding of your new veneers while you sleep.
- **Invisalign® Clear Braces:** Your new, clear braces will help straighten your teeth and give you the confidence you need to face the world with a brand new smile. But unlike veneers, they require a special set of cleaning instructions that your dentist should give you. Once a day, brush them with a soft toothbrush using cold or lukewarm water much as you would your own teeth. Invisalign offers a special cleaning system that can be ordered online to soak and clean your aligners as needed.
- **ZOOM!® Teeth Whitening:** To keep your teeth their brightest,

continue to clean your teeth much as you would previously: brushing twice a day and flossing regularly. An electric toothbrush is a powerful tool to help keep the stains away. Some people like baking soda or baking soda formula pastes to aid in stain removal. For regular touch-ups, your dental expert can provide you with Zoom! Weekender or Nite White gel.

- **Snap-On Smile®:** Caring for your Snap-On Smile® is truly a snap, but it requires one extra step to do so thoroughly. First, take off your appliance and clean your teeth as you normally would: brush and floss properly. Next, clean your appliance according to the proper care procedures prescribed by your dental expert. Your dentist should provide you with a special cleaning solution for your appliance and additional cleaning supplies can be ordered online at www.snaponsmile.com.
- **Tooth Colored Fillings:** Some people believe that once a filling is placed, they are safe from getting cavities in that tooth again. Unfortunately, this is not true! Cavities can still form under the margins of your fillings where the filling and tooth come together, so cleaning them as you always would by brushing and flossing regularly is crucial. Your dentist will also want to pay special attention to them during your routine, twice-yearly visits. A special note about brushing your porcelain fillings: many people brush only the front of their teeth. I recommend, in addition to brushing just the front of your teeth that you brush both the top of your teeth, biting surface and behind your teeth and continue to floss as well.
- **Dental Implants:** Treat your implants like your own teeth; care for them much as you would your own. Your dental expert will pay special attention to your periodontal care as well as your medical health to make sure that you have the proper amount of bone to support the implant.
- **Bonding:** While dental bonding quickly becomes part of your own teeth, there are a few special considerations to take when cleaning them. For starters, minimize or avoid consuming foods and beverages that can tarnish and stain the natural look that your dental professional worked so hard to achieve. Also,

be sure to use a soft brush head and brush thoroughly as well as floss between your teeth to avoid decay. If you grind your teeth at night or clench during the day, consider having a night guard made to protect your bonding from chipping off.

A-List Advice:

Please use this section as a supplement to the care instructions your dental expert gave you along with your A-List Smile. Procedures are continually updated and your dentist can provide you with the latest guidelines and routines to help care for your new smile.

What Next?

Caring for an A-List Smile does not end with brushing, flossing and regular trips to your dentist. It doesn't end with nutrition, healthy snacking or mouth guards. What's next for your new A-List Smile?

Depending on your product or procedure, you may need more routine dental visits than the standard "twice a year" recommendation. You should always check with your dentist before leaving his or her office as to how many visits you will need to maintain your new A-List Smile.

Thankfully, most dental professionals pay particular attention to aftercare and usually send you home with an armload of reading material to help you understand, care for and schedule routine visits for proper upkeep of your smile.

If you used a particularly busy or well-respected dental expert, find someone at the office – a hygienist, receptionist or assistant – who can be your "liaison" if you do end up having further questions about your new smile. It is always important to have a "go to" person in the office for just such occasions.

A-List Advice:

Make caring for your new smile as much of a priority as was getting your new smile. Most procedures are long-lasting, some are even permanent, IF you care for them properly. If not, you could be sporting a D-List smile sooner than you think!

Epilogue:

Fame Should Last Longer Than 15 Minutes – So Should Your Smile

"A smile is the universal welcome."

~ Max Eastman

Since having an A-List Smile is more than just a hobby for so many of my celebrity clients, I am eager to send readers from all walks of life away from this book with a positive mental image and a brighter, whiter smile. This Epilogue provides both a pat on the back and a kick in the pants; for those who have chosen to follow my advice and pursue an A-List Smile, there is a recap of what they can expect.

For those who are still on the fence, there is a brief section restating my point that "your mouth is your doorway to new friends, new experiences and a new you; don't close it before you have a chance to meet your destiny."

So, what does the future have in store for you and your new A-List Smile? Truthfully, the sky is the limit. Hopefully you realize the new lease on life your new smile has given you, and treat it with the proper care and respect it deserves. After all, smiling isn't just a gift we give ourselves; it's also a gift we give to others.

In addition to making you feel more confident, secure and satisfied, your new smile can:

- **Brighten a day**
- **Sympathize**
- **Turn a frown upside down**
- **Inspire**
- **Lift sagging spirits**
- **Motivate**
- **Share affection without a single word**
- **Encourage**

One thing I've noticed with my patients is that the more they show off their A-List smiles, the more pride they feel and the more likely they are to care for them properly. So, have you showed off your new smile yet? Not just to friends and family, but to everyone and anyone?

One of the most understated ways in which you can care for your new A-List Smile is to use it – often. Not only is smiling good for you (when in doubt, re-read Steps 1 and 2 of this book), but it's also addictive; so the more you smile, the more you want to smile.

Remember that brushing and flossing and routine dental visits, while crucial, are not the only ways to care for your new smile. The "use it or lose it" rule applies to your smile as well as your muscles.

After all, what good is an A-List Smile if nobody ever sees it?

A-List Advice:

You've worked hard to get an A-List Smile; now go forth and use it wisely, with confidence, style and grace that comes from the knowledge that you now have the smile you always wanted – and the confidence you deserve!

Your "Backstage Pass" to Dental Resources

A book designed to give you a Hollywood A-List Smile would be virtually incomplete without giving you a "backstage pass" to all the dental resources you'll need to make that dream a reality. In this section you will find a variety of resources, from other books on helping you achieve a beautiful smile to my Top-10 Dental Information Sites; it's all here, waiting for you to explore:

From the Bookshelf:
Other Recommended Titles for Beautifying Your Smile

- ***Billion Dollar Smile:*** *A Complete Guide to Your Extreme Smile Makeover* by Bill Dorfman (Thomas Nelson, 2006)
- ***Smile:*** *The Ultimate Guide to Achieving Smile Beauty* by Jonathan B. Levine and Jane Larkworthy (Wellness Central, 2006)
- ***Change Your Smile*** by Ronald E. Goldstein (Quintessence Publishing, 1997)
- ***The Perfect Smile:*** *The Complete Guide to Cosmetic Dentistry* by James Doundoulakis (Hatherleigh Press, 2002)

Dr. Austin's Top-10 Dental Information Sites

For all your dental information needs, I've gathered my Top-10 sites to help cut through the online clutter:

1. **American Academy of Cosmetic Dentistry (AACD):**
(http://www.aacd.com/public1/index.asp)

The American Academy of Cosmetic Dentistry has an incredible public section on their website for those who are looking to have the smile of their dreams, an A-List Smile. Here you can locate a cosmetic dentist in your area that has gone the extra mile in training in the latest cosmetic dentistry techniques, read patient smile makeover testimonies, view a gallery of before and after photos, and even watch videos of cosmetic dentists in action performing various smile makeovers.

2. **American Dental Association (ADA):**
(http://www.ada.org/public/index.asp)

The American Dental Association is one of the most trusted websites for dental health news and information for consumers and media. The ADA presents an A-Z index of dental topics and leaves no stone unturned. Find links to products that contain the ADA Seal, Dental FAQ's, oral health videos, and news releases.

3. **WebMD Health: Dental Health Center:**
(http://www.webmd.com/oral-health/)

This site offers hot topics on oral health, information on daily dental care, warning signs and symptoms of common dental problems as well as information on cosmetic dentistry. You will also find oral health blogs and a message board where you can chat with others about dental issues.

4. **Medline Plus: Dental Health:**
(http://www.nlm.nih.gov/medlineplus/dentalhealth.html)

Sponsored by the National Institute of Health (NIH) and the U.S National Library of Medicine, this site not only gives overviews on proper oral health and prevention, but offers information specific to men, women and seniors and their oral health. You will also find dental statistics, links to dental organizations and financial resources and interesting dental articles.

5. **Las Vegas Institute (LVI) Smile:**
(http://www.lvismile.com/lvismile/home.asp)

The Las Vegas Institute (LVI) is an advanced dental studies training center that trains dentists in excellence and beauty in cosmetic dentistry. This site offers contests to win a smile makeover, information on cosmetic dentistry, life changing testimonies, FAQ's and photos.

6. **American Dental Hygiene Association (ADHA):**
(http://www.adha.org/oralhealth/index.html)

The highlight of the American Dental Hygienists' Association website is the section called "Easy Instructions" which gives a fantastic visual demonstration along with instructions on the proper brushing and flossing techniques. You will also find fact sheets on various dental topics. This site contains Spanish language materials as well.

7. **About.com Dentistry**
(http://dentistry.about.com)

This website is very easy to navigate through as it offers interesting dental topics that are practical and current, contains blogs and offers information on dental conditions, treatment and prevention.

8. **Yahoo! Health: Oral Care Center**
(http://health.yahoo.com/oralcare/)

This site spotlights their top-5 popular dental topics. Find a host of oral care information as well. Readers vote on how helpful the articles are so you can gauge if you want to read them.

9. **Wikipedia: oral hygiene**
(http://en.wikipedia.org/wiki/Oral_hygiene)

This popular online encyclopedia offers great explanations in laymen's terms and photos on proper oral care. The site also reviews foods that are beneficial and harmful to the teeth, and reviews the links between oral health and systemic diseases such as heart attack, stroke, diabetes and osteoporosis.

10. **Healthy Teeth:**
(http://www.healthyteeth.org/tobacco/index.html)

This is an animated site designed to teach children and adults about proper dental hygiene. It's a great site to learn the basics about cavities, flossing, braces, nutrition and the negative effects of smoking.

Save More on Dental Products Through Shopping Online

Where can you get the latest dental care products, everything from denture care and dental floss to toothbrushes and toothpaste to mouthwash and whitening kits, online and up to half-price? The web can be a valuable tool when researching such products, but when it comes to buying them the experience is nothing short of A-List! Here are some of my seven favorite resources for securing great dental cleaning products online:

1. www.Drugstore.com: "Oral Care"
2. www.ShoppingYahoo.com: "Oral Care"
3. www.Shopping.com: "Oral Care"
4. www.Amazon.com: "Oral Hygiene"
5. www.CVS.com: "Oral Care"
6. www.Just4Teeth.com
7. www.Walgreens.com: "Mouth Care"

Free and/or Low-Cost Basic Care

The Centers for Medicare & Medicaid Services (CMS) administers three important federally-funded programs: Medicare, Medicaid and the State Children's Health Insurance Program (SCHIP).

Medicare is a health insurance program for people who are 65 years and older or for people with specific disabilities. Medicare does not cover most routine dental care or dentures. Visit http://www.cms.hhs.gov/MedicareDentalCoverage/.

Medicaid is a state-run program that provides medical benefits, and in some cases dental benefits, to eligible individuals and families. States set their own guidelines regarding who is eligible and what services are covered. Most states provide limited emergency dental services for people age 21 or over, while some offer comprehensive services. For most individuals under the age of 21, dental services are provided under Medicaid. Visit http://www.cms.hhs.gov/MedicaidDentalCoverage/.

SCHIP helps children up to age 19 who are without health insurance. SCHIP provides medical coverage and, in most cases, dental services to children who qualify. Dental services covered under this program vary from state to state. Visit http://www.cms.hhs.gov/SCHIPDentalCoverage/.

CMS can provide detailed information about each of these programs and refer you to state programs where applicable. If you currently have Medicare, call 1-800-MEDICARE (1-800-633-4227). Others may call 1-877-267-2323 or visit the CMS web site at http://www.cms.hhs.gov.

You can also write to them at the address below:

Centers for Medicare & Medicaid Services
7500 Security Boulevard
Baltimore, Maryland 21244

[**Source**: *NIH Publication No. 07-6097*]

Dental Schools (Take Two)

Below is a listing of all accredited dental education programs in the United States. Graduates receive either a DDS or DMD degree. Questions related to admission's criteria and application process should be directed to the dental school. [**Source**: *American Dental Association*]

AL

University of Alabama School of Dentistry at UAB
1530 3rd Avenue S.
SDB 406
Birmingham, AL 35294-0007
Dean: Dr. Huw F. Thomas
Phone: (205) 934-4720
Web Address: www.dental.uab.edu

AZ

A.T. Still University Arizona School of Dentistry and Oral Health
5850 East Still Circle
Mesa, AZ 85206
Dean: Dr. Jack Dillenberg
Phone: (480) 219-6000
Web Address: www.atsu.edu/asdoh

Midwestern University College of Dental Medicine
19555 North 59th Avenue
Glendale, AZ 85308
Dean: Dr. Richard J. Simonsen
Phone: 623/572-3800
Web Address: www.midwestern.edu

CA

Loma Linda University School of Dentistry
Dental School
Loma Linda, CA 92350
Dean: Dr. Charles J. Goodacre
Phone: (909) 558-4222
Web Address: www.llu.edu/llu/dentistry

University of California at Los Angeles School of Dentistry
Center for Health Science
Rm 53-038
Los Angeles, CA 90095-1668
Dean: Dr. No-Hee Park
Phone: (310) 206-6063
Web Address: www.dent.ucla.edu

University of California at San Francisco School of Dentistry
513 Parnassus Ave
S-630
San Francisco, CA 94143
Dean: Dr. John Featherstone
Phone: 415/476-1323
Web Address: www.dentistry.ucsf.edu/

University of Southern California School of Dentistry
925 W. 34th Street
Los Angeles, CA 90089-6041
Dean: Sigmund H. Abelson
Phone: (213) 740-3124
Web Address: www.usc.edu/hsc/dental

University of the Pacific Arthur A. Dugoni School of Dentistry
2155 Webster Street
San Francisco, CA 94115
Dean: Dr. Patrick J. Ferrillo Jr.
Phone: (415) 929-6425
Web Address: dental.pacific.edu

CO

University of Colorado Denver
School of Dental Medicine; Lazzara Center for Oral-Facial Health
13065 E. 17th Avenue
Aurora, CO 80045
Dean: Dr. Denise K. Kassebaum

Phone: (303) 724-7100
Web Address: www.uchsc.edu/sod

CT

University of Connecticut School of Dental Medicine
263 Farmington Avenue
Farmington, CT 06030-3915
Dean: Dr. R.(Monty) Lamont MacNeil
Phone: (860) 679-2808
Web Address: www.sdm.uchc.edu

DC

Howard University College of Dentistry
600 "W" Street, N.W.
Washington, DC 20059
Dean: Dr. Leo E. Rouse
Phone: (202) 806-0440
Web Address: www.howard.edu

FL

Nova Southeastern University College of Dental Medicine
3200 S. University Drive
Fort Lauderdale, FL 33328
Dean: Dr. Robert A. Uchin
Phone: (954) 262-7311
Web Address: www.dental.nova.edu
University of Florida College of Dentistry
1600 SW Archer Rd.
Rm D4-6
Gainesville, FL 32610-0405
Dean: Dr. Teresa A. Dolan
Phone: (352) 273-5802
Web Address: www.dental.ufl.edu

GA

Medical College of Georgia School of Dentistry
1120 15th Street
Rm AD 1119
Augusta, GA 30912-0200
Dean: Dr. Connie L. Drisko
Phone: (706) 721-2117
Web Address: www.mcg.edu/SOD

IA

University of Iowa College of Dentistry
100 Dental Science Bldg.
Iowa City, IA 52242
Dean: Dr. David C. Johnsen
Phone: (319) 335-7144 or 45
Web Address: www.dentistry.uiowa.edu

IL

Southern Illinois University School of Dental Medicine
2800 College Avenue
Bldg 273/2300
Alton, IL 62002
Dean: Dr. Ann M. Boyle
Phone: (618) 474-7120
Web Address: www.siue.edu/sdm/

University of Illinois at Chicago College of Dentistry
801 South Paulina Street
Suite # 102
Chicago, IL 60612
Dean: Dr. Bruce S. Graham
Phone: (312) 996-1040
Web Address: www.dentistry.uic.edu

IN

Indiana University School of Dentistry
1121 West Michigan Street
Indianapolis, IN 46202
Dean: Dr. Lawrence Goldblatt
Phone: (317) 274-7461
Web Address: www.iusd.iupui.edu/default.aspx

KY

University of Kentucky College of Dentistry
800 Rose Street
D 136 UKMC
Lexington, KY 40536-0297
Dean: Dr. Sharon P. Turner
Phone: (859) 323-1884
Web Address: www.mc.uky.edu/Dentistry

University of Louisville School of Dentistry
501 S. Preston Street
Louisville, KY 40292
Dean: Dr. John J. Sauk
Phone: 502/852-5295
Web Address: www.dental.louisville.edu/dental

LA

Louisiana State University School of Dentistry
1100 Florida Avenue
New Orleans, LA 70119-2799
Dean: Dr. Henry Gremillion
Phone: 504-619-8500
Web Address: www.lsusd.lsuhsc.edu

MA

Boston University Goldman School of Dental Medicine
100 East Newton Street
Boston, MA 02118
Dean: Dr. Jeffrey W. Hutter
Phone: 617-638-4780
Web Address: www.dentalschool.bu.edu

Harvard University School of Dental Medicine
188 Longwood Avenue
Boston, MA 02115
Dean: Dr. R. Bruce Donoff
Phone: (617) 432-1401
Web Address: www.hsdm.med.harvard.edu

Tufts University School of Dental Medicine
One Kneeland Street
Boston, MA 02111
Dean: Dr. Lonnie H. Norris
Phone: (617) 636-6636
Web Address: www.tufts.edu/dental

MD

University of Maryland Baltimore College of Dental Surgery
650 W. Baltimore Street
Suite 6402
Baltimore, MD 21201
Dean: Dr. Christian S. Stohler
Phone: (410) 706-7461
Web Address: www.dental.umaryland.edu

MI

University of Detroit Mercy School of Dentistry
2700 Martin Luther King Jr. Blvd
(MB 98)
Detroit, MI 48208-2576
Dean: Dr. Mert N. Aksu
Phone: (313) 494-6621
Web Address: www.udmercy.edu/dental

University of Michigan School of Dentistry
1011 N. University Ave.
Ann Arbor, MI 48109-1078
Dean: Dr. Peter J. Polverini
Phone: (734) 763-3311/3111
Web Address: www.dent.umich.edu

MN

University of Minnesota School of Dentistry
Room 15-209 Moos Tower
515 S.E. Delaware Street
Minneapolis, MN 55455
Dean: Dr. Patrick M. Lloyd
Phone: (612) 625-9982
Web Address: www.dentistry.umn.edu/

MO

University of Missouri-Kansas City School of Dentistry
650 East 25th Street
Kansas City, MO 64108
Dean: Dr. Nancy Mills
Phone: 816-235-2010
Web Address: www.umkc.edu/dentistry

MS

University of Mississippi School of Dentistry
Medical Center;
2500 North State Street
Jackson, MS 39216-4505
Dean: Dr. Buford O. Gilbert
Phone: (601) 984-6125
Web Address: www.dentistry.umc.edu

NC

University of North Carolina School of Dentistry
UNC-CH CB# 7450
1090 Old Dental Bldg
Chapel Hill, NC 27599-7450
Dean: Dr. John N. Williams
Phone: (919) 966-2731
Web Address: www.dent.unc.edu

NE

Creighton University School of Dentistry
2500 California Plaza
Omaha, NE 68178-0240
Dean: Dr. Steven W. Friedrichsen
Phone: (402) 280-5060
Web Address: www.cudental.creighton.edu

University of Nebraska Medical Center College of Dentistry
40th & Holdrege Streets
Lincoln, NE 68583-0740
Dean: Dr. John W. Reinhardt
Phone: (402) 472-1344
Web Address: www.unmc.edu/dentistry

NJ

University of Medicine & Dentistry of New Jersey
New Jersey Dental School
110 Bergen St.;
Room B815
Newark, NJ 07103-2425
Dean: Dr. Cecile A. Feldman
Phone: (973) 972-4633
Web Address: www.dentalschool.umdnj.edu/

NV

University of Nevada Las Vegas School of Dental Medicine
Shadow Lane Campus
1001 Shadow Lane
Las Vegas, NV 89106-4124
Dean: Dr. Karen P. West
Phone: (702) 774-2500
Web Address: www.dentalschool.unlv.edu/

NY

Columbia University College of Dental Medicine
630 West 168th Street
PH7 East Room 122
New York, NY 10032
Dean: Dr. Ira B. Lamster
Phone: (212) 305-4511
Web Address: www.cpmcnet.columbia.edu/dept/dental

New York University College of Dentistry
345 East 24th Street
New York, NY 10010
Dean: Dr. Charles N Bertolami
Phone: 212/998-9898
Web Address: www.nyu.edu/dental/

State University of New York at Buffalo School of Dental Medicine
325 Squire Hall;
3435 Main Street
Buffalo, NY 14214-3008
Dean: Dr. Richard N. Buchanan
Phone: (716) 829-2836
Web Address: www.sdm.buffalo.edu

State University of New York at Stony Brook School of Dental Medicine
Health Sciences Center;
154 Rockland Hall
Stony Brook, NY 11794-8700
Dean: Dr. Lorne Golub
Phone: 631-632-8990
Web Address: www.hsc.stonybrook.edu/dental

OH

Case Western Reserve Univ. School of Dental Medicine
10900 Euclid Avenue
Cleveland, OH 44106-4905
Dean: Dr. Jerold S. Goldberg
Phone: (216) 368-3266
Web Address: www.case.edu/dental/site/main.html

Ohio State University College of Dentistry
305 West 12th Avenue;
PO Box 182357
Columbus, OH 43218-2357
Dean: Dr. Carole A. Anderson
Phone: 614-292-9750
Web Address: www.dent.ohio-state.edu

OK

University of Oklahoma College of Dentistry
1201 N. Stonewall Avenue
Oklahoma City, OK 73117
Dean: Dr. Stephen K. Young
Phone: (405)271-6326 or5444
Web Address: www.dentistry.ouhsc.edu

OR

Oregon Health and Science University School of Dentistry
611 SW Campus Drive
Portland, OR 97239
Dean: Dr. Jack W. Clinton
Phone: (503) 494-8801
Web Address: www.ohsu.edu/sod/admissions

PA

Temple University The Maurice H. Kornberg School of Dentistry
3223 North Broad Street
Philadelphia, PA 19140
Dean: Dr. Amid I. Ismail
Phone: 215-707-2799
Web Address: www.temple.edu/dentistry

University of Pennsylvania School of Dental Medicine
240 South 40th Street;
Robert Shattner Center
Philadelphia, PA 19104-6030
Dean: Dr. Thomas P. Sollecito
Phone: 215-898-8941
Web Address: www.dental.upenn.edu

University of Pittsburgh School of Dental Medicine
3501 Terrace Street
Pittsburgh, PA 15261
Dean: Dr. Thomas W. Braun
Phone: (412) 648-1938
Web Address: www.dental.pitt.edu

PR

University of Puerto Rico School of Dental Medicine
Medical Sciences Campus
Main Building-Office #A103B, 1st Floor
San Juan, PR 00936-5067
Dean: Dr. Yilda M. Rivera
Phone: (787) 758-2525 x1105
Web Address: www.dental.rcm.upr.edu/

SC

Medical University of South Carolina College of Dental Medicine
171 Ashley Avenue;
PO Box 250507
Charleston, SC 29425-1376
Dean: Dr. John J. Sanders
Phone: (843) 792-3811
Web Address: www.gradstudies.musc.edu/dentistry/dental.html

TN

Meharry Medical College School of Dentistry
1005 D.B. Todd Blvd.
Nashville, TN 37208
Dean: Dr. William B. Butler
Phone: (615) 327-6207
Web Address: www.dentistry.mmc.edu

University of Tennessee College of Dentistry
University of Tennessee Health Science Ctr;
875 Union Avenue
Memphis, TN 38163
Dean: Dr. Mark Patters
Phone: 901/448-6202
Web Address: www.utmem.edu/dentistry

TX

Baylor College of Dentistry Component of Texas A & M Health Sci Ctr
3302 Gaston Avenue
Dallas, TX 75246
Dean: Dr. James S. Cole
Phone: (214) 828-8201
Web Address: www.tambcd.edu

Univ. of Texas Hlth Science Cnt-Houston Dental Branch
6516 M. D. Anderson Blvd.;
Room 147;
Houston, TX 77225-0068
Dean: Dr. Catherine M. Flaitz
Phone: (713) 500-4021
Web Address: www.db.uth.tmc.edu

University of Texas Hlth Science Cnt-San Antonio Dental School
7703 Floyd Curl Drive
Mail Code 7914
San Antonio, TX 78284-7914
Dean: Dr. Kenneth L. Kalkwarf
Phone: (210) 567-3160
Web Address: www.dental.uthscsa.edu

VA

Virginia Commonwealth University School of Dentistry
P.O. Box 980566
520 North 12th Street
Richmond, VA 23298-0566
Dean: Dr. Ronald J. Hunt
Phone: (804) 827-2077
Web Address: www.dentistry.vcu.edu

WA

University of Washington-Health Sciences School of Dentistry
D322 Health Sciences Bldg.;
1959 NE Pacific St.;
Seattle, WA 98195
Dean: Dr. Martha J. Somerman
Phone: (206) 543-5982
Web Address: www.dental.washington.edu

WI

Marquette University School of Dentistry
1801 W. Wisconsin Avenue
Milwaukee, WI 53233
Dean: Dr. William Keith Lobb
Phone: (414) 288-7485
Web Address: www.dental.mu.edu

WV

West Virginia University School of Dentistry
Robert C. Byrd Health Sci Ctr.;
1150 HSC North/Medical Center Drive;
Morgantown, WV 26506-9400
Dean: Dr. Louise T. Veselicky
Phone: 304/293-2521
Web Address: www.hsc.wvu.edu/sod

Photo credits:

Susan Goode Estep, DMD, FACE
Atlanta Dental Spa
1875 Old Alabama Road
Suite 130
Roswell, GA 30076
(770) 998-3838
www.AtlantaDentalSpa.com

* * * * *

Peter D. Boulden, DMD, FACE
Atlanta Dental Spa
1875 Old Alabama Road
Suite 130
Roswell, GA 30076
(770) 998-3838
www.AtlantaDentalSpa.com

* * * * *

Robert J. Gallien, DDS
4620 Hwy 58
Chattanooga, TN 37416
(423) 894-57
www.SmileChattanooga.com

* * * * *

Ira Handschuh, DDS
The Dental Design Center
280 Dobbs Ferry Road
White Plains , N.Y. 10956
(914)683-5898
www.dentaldesigncenter.com

* * * * *

Dental Associates of CT
36 Padanaram Road
Danbury, CT 06811
(203) 730-1267
www.DentalAssociates.us

* * * * *

Dr. Eric McRory, DDS
Northside Dental Care
3031 Orleans Street, Suite 201, Bellingham, WA.
Phone: 360-676-1138
http://northsidedentalcare.net

* * * * *

Dr. Marc Liechtung, DMD
Snap On Smile
462 Seventh Avenue
19th Floor
New York, NY 10018

About the Author:

Dr. Catrise Austin

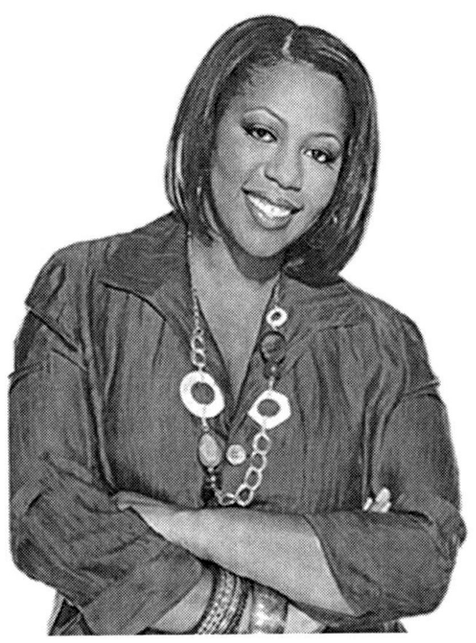

*"With **5 Steps to a Hollywood A-list Smile**, Dr. Catrise Austin has unveiled her years of brilliant dentistry work mixed with serious marketing savvy and a compelling personal narrative that brings to life why healthy teeth matter. Not only will you want to have an Oscar-winning smile, but you will also appreciate that self-esteem boost Dr. Austin is equally adept at providing in this great read."*

~ Kevin Powell

What started out as a routine visit to the dentist changed a young lady's life and her future.

"I never felt confident about my teeth. I never liked the look of my smile." Young Catrise Austin thought she would be stuck forever, hiding behind a smile that didn't make her feel pretty or confident. She thought that she was simply going to have to live life with what she was given. However, a routine "dental experience," as she calls it, changed her forever.

Inspired, Catrise completed her undergraduate studies at the

University of Michigan, majoring in psychology. She wisely believed that understanding the emotional impact of dentistry on her patients was as important as mastering the necessary medical knowledge. Her intuition proved to be beneficial as her clinical interaction during her second portion of dental school went so well that she completed her requirements early and created an award winning senior presentation on HIV in the Mid-life and Elderly Population.

A great deal of Dr. Austin's relaxation time was spent in New York City upon graduating from Dental School and it was during this time Dr. Austin met Tracey Morgan, Mike Epps, Dave Chappelle, and other up and coming comedians as she frequented The Boston Comedy Club.

In the midst of her celebrity-driven downtime, she had an epiphany: that's when the "Dentist to the Stars" was born. "I knew that they had to have the best smiles of all and after realizing that I couldn't work for someone and be as successful as I had envisioned, I knew I had to start my own practice."

Describing herself as self-motivated, Dr. Austin found herself acquiring much her clientele from record labels, comedy clubs, and other New York hot spots. Because of her prime location, she was exposed to many celebrity clients who heard that "The Dentist to the Stars" was doing great things with smiles.

But beyond the celebrated elite, Dr. Austin's true goal is to empower and educate ALL about the importance of dental health, oral hygiene. "The benefits are a blessing, but my motivation is to make people be their best." Her commitment to her patients is exemplary. "I don't double-book and my appointments are at least an hour. When I schedule time for you, it is a reservation! It's not a rushed environment. Every patient gets their deserved time. I would not be able to deliver the care I do with just 30 minutes."

Dr. Austin purposed having an office of VIP proportions located on the opulent and populated 57th Street in Manhattan and not a clinic. "I try to undo the horror stories that people have about the dentist." Further, she is compassionate in her concern for patients, understanding that many people are stuck in a period when the dentist's office wasn't as advanced as it is now.

Dr. Austin often shares her own story with her patients, so that they know that she understands their fears, but *really* understands their desires and the issues that an uncomfortable smile can reveal. Lastly, popular makeover shows airing today show regular people who, with a productive trip to the dentist, can regain and revive long-lost self-esteem. "The internet has helped a great deal to show people that the dentist's office can change your life and your smile," says Dr. Austin.

Just ask a young shining star named Catrise.

Free bonus offer for
5 Steps to a Hollywood A-List Smile

Here's your chance to get a sneak preview of how you too can have a Hollywood A-List Smile!

Send us a close up "before" photo of your smile and we'll send you a digital computer simulated "after" photo of your Hollywood smile makeover for **FREE** (a $150 value) compliments of Hollywood Dental Smile Studio of Hollywood, California.

Before

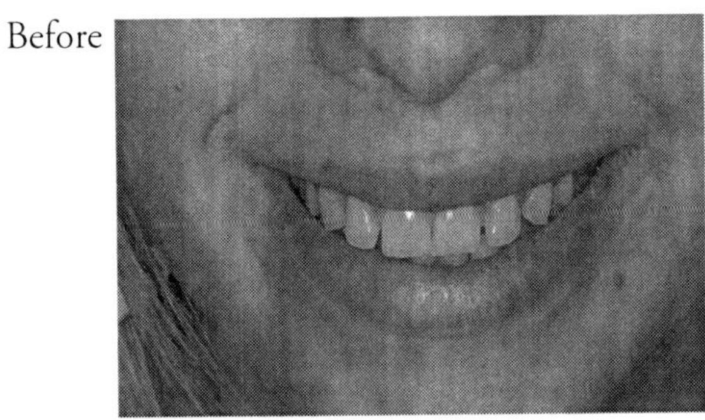

After

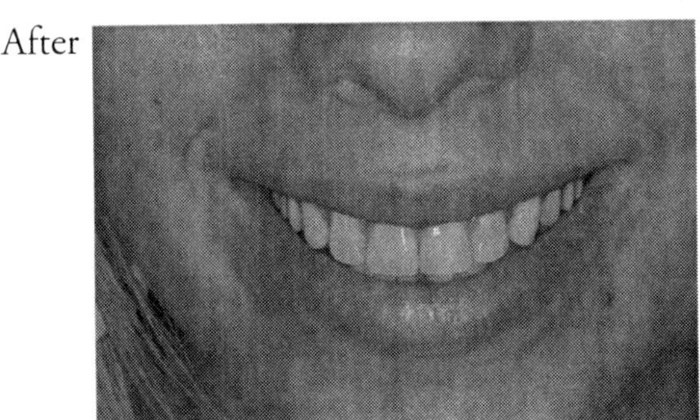

To redeem your FREE bonus, visit our website
www.hollywoodalistsmiles.com

LaVergne, TN USA
06 October 2009

160097LV00004B/150/P

9 781600 376443